Tomas Silber M.D. editor

ETHICAL ISSUES IN THE TREATMENT OF CHILDREN AND ADOLESCENTS

SLACK

Printed in the United States of America

Library of Congress Catalog Card Number: 83-050283

ISBN: 0-943432-08-1

Published by: SLACK Incorporated
6900 Grove Rd.
Thorofare, NJ 08086

Last digit is print number: 8 7 6 5 4 3 2 1

To Our Children

Contents

SECTION FOUR: SPECIAL PROBLEMS

SECTION FIVE: EXPERIMENTATION WITH CHILDREN

SECTION SIX: SOCIETY AND CHILDREN

Foreword

One of my early internships was with the section of pediatric surgery of Cornell Medical College. Cornell, at that time, had an affiliation with St. Mary's Hospital for Children situated in the lower portion of "Hell's Kitchen" in New York City.

One day a badly deformed newborn baby girl was brought to the hospital. She had a hare-lip and cleft palate, a right eye socket without an eye, a small lump of flesh instead of the right ear, and stumps for the right arm and right leg. The infant came from the slum area in the neighborhood.

When the baby was six days old she developed a severe diarrhea and dehydration. Should we save the baby? I went to the Sister Superior of the hospital. "Sister," I said, "This terribly deformed baby girl comes from a very poor, underprivileged and uneducated family. She has no chance for happiness in this world. She will have only the pain of numerous operations with questionable results. Now the child has a severe diarrhea and dehydration. I believe this may be God's way of taking this unfortunate infant out of the world. Will you permit me not to treat this baby vigorously?"

Old Sister Catherine rose up from her desk, gave me a strong stare for a moment and said something I'll never forget. "Dr. Levine, who do you think you are—God?"

So we treated the infant vigorously, and she recovered. And she started on her long series of reparative operations—and a pathetic future.

Often through the years, when I have met with serious moral and ethical problems in my pediatric practice, I have thought of Sister Catherine—but at times when in a severe dilemma I have felt that I was acting not as God but with God and for God.

All of us who have practiced pediatrics for any length of time are not infrequently confronted by ethical problems. And often arriving at a decision in such cases is most difficult.

Furthermore, in considering moral and ethical problems there is an area often overlooked—legal responsibility. I recently received a copy of the newspaper *Counsel*, published by the legal counsellors of the Children's Hospital—National Medical Center in Washington, D.C. In this issue three cases are reviewed in which physicians were sued by parents.

The first case was that of a child born with polycystic kidneys. The child died and their physician assured the parents that the condition was not hereditary. So the mother became pregnant again and the next child also had polycystic kidneys and died in two-and-one-half years. The second case was that of a 37-year-old mother who had a child born with Down's syndrome. She had not been told of the availability of amniocentesis with the opportunity of terminating the pregnancy if the fetal cells showed evidence of the condition. The third case was that of a child with Tay-Sachs disease born to parents of Eastern European Jewish extraction. Blood tests can detect carriers and amniocentesis can give evidence if the fetus has inherited the disease. At no time were the parents told of the link between their heritage and the disease—nor were they told that the disease could be detected by amniocentesis, and pregnancy terminated.

All of these parents sued their physicians—and in all three cases the physician lost. The article notes that the physician's personal feelings as to the risks involved in testing, or the morality of abortions, must not enter into the counselling process.

Several important facts have been learned as a result of numerous malpractice suits. First, the pediatrician or obstetrician must always tell the parents the legal medical opportunities open to them. Secondly, if a physician decides on what he considers an ethical course, he must first inform the parents and gain their consent.

We should realize that one cannot present a set of rules to cover all ethical problems. What may be advisable in one case may not be in another. So much depends on the particular situation, the parents' feelings, the age of the child, the religious beliefs and the laws of the area.

However, the material in this book should be of the greatest interest and value to all involved in the physical, mental, and emotional care of children.

We are all essentially dedicated not only to bringing up healthy and happy children but also to giving them the best world possible to live in. But each of us has his or her own moral and ethical beliefs and feelings which may color our outlook on child care.

This book, presented by Dr. Tomas J. Silber and his contributors, should aid greatly in clarifying our viewpoint on these many and complicated subjects.

Milton I. Levine, MD
New York, NY

Foreword

This work breaks new ground for the field of medical ethics. While there exist clinical textbooks on pediatric and adolescent medicine, we have not yet had an ethics book that covers the first major part of the life span—the period from birth to the completion of adolescence.

The essays collected in this anthology cover a broad range of topics. The primary focus is, as it should be, on the clinical relationship among minors, parents, and health professionals. Yet the important topic of research involving children is not neglected. A final, intriguing part of this volume explores the relationship to social institutions, including health care institutions. Here one sees the field of medical ethics breaking beyond its traditional boundaries to examine questions about the social context in which patients live and health professionals practice.

Great care has obviously been employed in selecting the essays to be included in this work. The essays are relatively brief, clearly written, and concrete in their use of case materials and examples. The content of all the essays will be readily accessible to parents, to health professionals, and to philosophers and theologians who specialize in ethics.

Two major themes permeate this work. The first is the cluster of issues surrounding genetic defects, chromosomal abnormalities, and mental retardation. Decisions can now be made *about* individuals afflicted with these conditions from the earliest point at which prenatal diagnosis can be performed—we are fast moving toward first-trimester diagnosis of some conditions—to the end of adolescence. Decisions can be made *by* the mildly or moderately retarded and the genetically handicapped from the stage at which they are able to accept a measure of responsibility for their own futures. Whereas these decisions were at one time made privately—or, in the case of decisions by affected individuals, not allowed to be made at all—there is increasing interest within American society in having such decisions made in an explicit way, using generally accepted ethical standards that are subject to public review and scrutiny.

A second major theme that binds together the various parts of this fascinating book is the appropriate roles of children and adults in decisions about clinical care and participation in biomedical research. Here there is increasing acceptance of a developmental spectrum, of a gradual evolution in the child's ability to take responsibility for his or her decisions. There is also increasing recognition of various spheres of life or areas of competence. From this view, a 13-year-old might be perfectly capable of making decisions about schooling but unable, as yet, to manage his or her financial affairs. Such nuances in the decision-making abilities of minors are not easily incorporated into public policy. There, global transitions at age 7 or 12 seem to provide clear guidance for administrators. However, the increasing recognition of individual differences in development of the diverse spheres of minors' activities constitutes a clear rationale for moving toward greater flexibility and individualization in the formulation of guidelines for minors' decision-making.

One hopes that this pioneering book will receive the wide reading it deserves and that it will contribute to the understanding and humane treatment of children and adolescents.

LeRoy Walters, PhD
Center for Bioethics
Kennedy Institute for Ethics
Georgetown University
Washington, DC

Introduction

Bioethics and the Treatment of Children

The contemporary interest in bioethics is the result of progress in medicine.[1] In the past, for example, there was no need for a physician to consider the concept of death: there was but one death. This has changed with the advent of new techniques that have made it possible to sustain life, or at least to sustain living matter. Terminology itself has become a problem; we must now make a distinction between human life, living matter, and persons. Doctors everywhere are now facing philosophical problems such as defining personhood and conceptualizing death. Many questions are also raised by the possibility of genetic screening, abortion, and complex technological interventions. All these issues clearly relate to decision-making.

Pediatricians and other professionals caring for children are deeply involved in these complex ethical situations and are constantly confronted with moral problems. Amniocentesis and abortion for genetic indications; treatment versus nontreatment in intensive care nurseries; problems of consent and confidentiality in the treatment of adolescent patients; and the morality of research with children are but a few examples of the dilemmas faced. The way these issues are confronted depends on one's understanding of medical ethics.

The term "medical ethics" is used in a variety of ways. In its narrowest sense, it refers to a body of codes of conduct developed by the medical profession. The Hippocratic oath is an example of its ancient origins, and the modern codes of organizations such as the American Health Association and the World Medical Association illustrate its continuity. This aspect of medical ethics promulgates the concept that medical ethics is restricted to what is thought and practiced by health professionals.[2]

Medical ethics in a wider sense is bioethics. That is: a systematic reflection on what is right and wrong in the practice of medicine.[3] This has always been a major theme in the Jewish and Christian traditions and is also expressed by the modern humanistic-philosophical approach.

A single conflict has characterized the field of medical ethics throughout its history: the tension between laypersons and physicians relating to decision-making. This has often been alluded to as "the universal-professional dichotomy."[4] This conflict can be resolved if one thinks of the "medical ethic" not as a special professional ethic, but rather as the specific application of a universal norm of ethical action. This solution has been voiced persuasively by Veatch, who goes as far as to say that the professional codes of medical ethics, "are actually dangerous diversions which lead professionals to believe that there is a special type of ethics appropriate for their own professional discipline." He proposed, "We must first reject the fallacy of generalization of expertise—that expertise about the technical facts of a given area also gives one expertise in the evaluation factor required for decision-making in that area. . ."[4] Thus, bioethics may be considered a discipline in which the field of universal ethics is applied to medicine. In other words, the moral problems involved in medical care are too important to be left to doctors alone.

Doctors treating children still have a lot to offer. Ramsey understands this well when he states, "For all the moral crisis in medical practice and in our civilization, generally, I myself would still trust 'the ethical physician' to discern the issues we face as well as or better than some overawed, excessively scientifically minded member of 'the public.' To say this is not 'the fallacy of generalization of expertise.' It is simple to say that to whom more is given of facing birth and death and pain and suffering in between, of him more is required in moral discernment in an age when that no longer flows from the decencies of one moral universe or the religious faith in which men formerly lived."[5] It is within that context that many pediatricians have developed and contributed their thoughts and reflections in this area.[6-10]

The contributions of ethicists and theologians trying to solve ethical problems in the treatment of children have also been remarkable. Yet, at times, we are concerned with the absence of these professionals from our daily lives. For example, serious ethical dilemmas are encountered every day in the intensive care nursery. In order to balance alternative consequences, an ethicist needs to understand the meaning of a diagnosis, the therapeutic tools involved, the prognosis, and so forth. Ethicists who have never been in an intensive care nursery lose an important dimension that could have enriched the data base on which they make many ethical judgments. Conversely, in an increasingly secularized culture, where as professionals we are being pressured into being only scientists, we can enrich our judgments with the experience brought about by familiarity with the concepts developed by ethicists and theologians.

Practitioners of bioethics coming from diverse backgrounds have a fascinating task: Physicians have to submerge themselves in the adventure of learning philosophical and theological work, while the philosopher and theologian have to emerge into the world of medicine, illness, and hospitals. The present generation of ethicists, perhaps *because* of their different professional origins, are enriching the discipline. This can be seen in the variety of approaches to main topics. For example, we physicians enjoy working on the specific problems we confront. This leads us to study the ethics of issues such as the physician/patient relationship and the withdrawal of treatment from the severely impaired newborn. The ethicists, on the other hand, focus their efforts on philosophically inspired taxonomy.[11] Thus, they concentrate their efforts on areas such as rights, justice, responsibility, and personhood. The theologians focus their attention on death and dying, human subject experimentation, and fetal research. In doing so, they introduce thought-provoking religious concepts, such as Ramsey's view of medical care as a sacred convenant between physicians and patients.[12]

Historical contingencies may speed up or slow down the development of bioethics. This field is not only under the influence of medicine, its traditions, and its developments, but it is also affected by other changing forces such as economic conditions, public reputation, political ideologies, and economic growth. These forces not only control resources, but they also determine the climate for growth. This, external circumstances influence the interests and theoretical preoccupations of bioethicists by contributing to their "Zeitgeist."[13]

It is the success of medicine that generates the new issues challenging all bioethicists. The search for answers to complex new medical problems forces us to look again into the meaning of basic human experiences. Inherent to the subject is a requirement for crossing disciplinary lines in the search for broader and deeper overall synthesis. It is a task for more than one generation. Pediatricians and advocates of children and youth have an important role to play, through personal reflections and through the input of their organizations. It is within this spirit that this book presents an anthology of classic and new contributions to elucidate the ethical problems encountered in pediatric practice. It gathers the efforts of physicians caring for children and adolescents, neonatologists, general pediatricians, practitioners of adolescent medicine, pediatric subspecialists, child advocates, ethicists, theologians, and lawyers, all expressed in the following pages as a testimony to the serious preoccupation and action that the issues merit.

Finally, I would like to acknowledge the teachers that allowed me to pursue this vocation at the Program in Special Studies of George Washington University, the visiting Scholar Program of the Joseph and Rose Kennedy Institute for Ethics of Georgetown University, and the moral support from Children's Hospital National Medical Center, and the dedicated aid given by Linda Harteker and Betsy Covel.

REFERENCES

1. Kass R: The New Biology: What Price Reliving Man's Estate? Science, Nov 19, 1971, pp 779–788.
2. Jonsen R, Hellegers Andre E: Conceptual Foundations for Ethics of Medical Care. *In* Tancredi LR (ed): Ethics of Health Care. National Academy of Science, 1974, pp 3–20.
3. Walters L: Bioethics as a Field of Ethics. *In* Beauchamp and Walters:

Contemporary Issues in Bioethics. California, Dickenson Publishing Co, 1978, pp 49–51.

4. Veatch RM: Medical Ethics: Professional or Universal? Harvard Theolog Rev 65:531–559, 1972.
5. Ramsey P: The Nature of Medical Ethics. *In* Veatch et al (eds): The Teaching of Medical Ethics. Hastings on Hudson, New York, Institute of Society, Ethics and the Life Sciences, 1971, pp 14–28.
6. Fost N: Ethical issues in the treatment of critically ill newborns. Pediatr Ann 10:383, 1981.
7. Cooke R: Ethics in Behalf of the Mentally Retarded Person. Pediatr Ann 10:390, 1981.
8. Silber T: Ethical Considerations in the Medical Care of Adolescents and Their Parents. Pediatr Ann 10:481, 1981.
9. Leikin S: Ethical Issues in Pediatric Hematology. Pediatr Ann 10:401, 1981.
10. Fleischman A: Teaching Medical Ethics in the Pediatric Training Program. Pediatr Ann 10:411, 1981.
11. Gorovits S: Moral Problems in Medicine. Englewood Cliffs, NJ, Prentice Hall, Inc, 1971, p 1.
12. Ramsey P: The Patient as a Person. New Haven, CT, Yale University Press, 1970.
13. Silber TJ: Bioethics, an Interdisciplinary Enterprise. J Rel Health, 21:21, 1982.

Contributors

CONSTANCE U. BATTLE MD, Medical Director and Chief Executive Officer, Hospital for Sick Children, Washington, DC; Professor of Child Health and Development, George Washington University School of Medicine, Washington, DC.

HOWARD BRODY MD, PhD, Assistant Professor of Family Practice and Philosophy, and Assistant Coordinator, Medical Humanities Program, Michigan State University, East Lansing, MI.

DANIEL CALLAHAN PhD, Director, Institute of Society, Ethics, and the Life Sciences, The Hastings Center, Hasting-On-Hudson, NY.

JEAN E. CARLIN MD, PhD, Director of Residency Training Program, Department of Psychiatry and Behavioral Sciences, College of Medicine, The University of Oklahoma, OK.

ROBERT E. COOKE MD, A. Conger Goodyear Professor of Pediatrics, State University of New York at Buffalo; Medical Director, Robert Warner Rehabilitation Center of the Children's Hospital of Buffalo; Chairman of the Scientific Advisory Board, Joseph P. Kennedy, Jr. Foundation.

C. RICHARD CORNELIUS JD, General Counsel, Children's Hospital National Medical Center, Washington, DC.

JULIAN B. FERHOLT MD, Associate Clinical Professor of Pediatrics/Psychiatry, Yale Child Study Center, Yale University, New Haven, CT.

NORMAN FOST MD, MPH, Professor, Department of Pediatrics and History of Medicine, Director, Program in Medical Ethics, University of Wisconsin School of Medicine, Madison, WI.

LYNN GORDON MS, Masters Program, Special Education Early Childhood Education, Former Director, Child Life Program, University of Maryland Hospital, Baltimore, MD.

ANGELA HOLDER LLM, Counsel for Medical Legal Affairs, Clinical Professor of Pediatrics (Law), Yale University, New Haven, CT.

ALBERT R. JONSEN PhD, Professor, Ethics in Medicine, Department of Medicine, University of California, San Francisco, CA.

SUSAN KLEINBERG MA, Director of Child Life Education, Mount Washington Pediatric Hospital, Inc., Baltimore, MD.

SANFORD R. LEIKIN MD, Chairman of the Department of Hematology/Oncology, Children's Hospital National Medical Center; Professor, Department of Child Health and Development, George Washington University School of Medicine, Washington, DC.

NANCY M. MANN MSW, Social Worker, Private Practice, Madison, CT.

MARY E. McCARTHY PhD, Faculty Research Associate, Institute for Child Study, College of Education, University of Maryland, College Park, MD.

JOSEPH NOSHPITZ MD, Senior Attending Staff Psychiatrist, Department of Psychiatry, Children's Hospital National Medical Center; Professor of Psychiatry and Behavioral Sciences and of Child Health and Development. George Washington University School of Medicine, Washington, DC.

MICHAEL ROTHENBERG MD, Professor of Psychiatry and Pediatrics, University of Washington School of Medicine; Head of Pediatric Liaison Division, Department of Child Psychiatry and Behavioral Medicine, Children's Orthopedic Hospital and Medical Center, Seattle, WA.

JOHN E. SCHOWALTER MD, Chief of Child Psychiatry, Professor of Pediatrics, Child Study Center, Yale University, New Haven, CT.

TOMAS J. SILBER MD, MASS, Director, Ambulatory Services, Adolescent and Young Adult Medicine, Children's Hospital National Medical Center; Associate Professor of Child Health and Development, George Washington University School of Medicine, Washington, DC.

WILLIAM A. SILVERMAN MD, former Professor of Pediatrics, College of Physicians and Surgeons, Columbia University, Christensen Visting Fellow, St. Catherine's College, University of Oxford, England.

SECTION ONE

GENETICS

Pediatricians historically have had a long-standing interest in preventive medicine. This has been extended to the field of genetics. In the 1980s, especially in developed countries, the impact of genetic defects has been impressive: approximately 2300 genetically related disorders have been identified. In some cases, an early diagnosis may assist in the treatment, as with phenylketonuria; in others, there is still little that can be done, as illustrated by Down's syndrome. Our ability to diagnose hereditary disorders and identify them prenatally raises new philosophical questions that require reflection and thoughtful action.

In this section, Daniel Callahan looks at broad issues raised by our new technology. He analyzes the concept of genetic abnormality and shows how it may presuppose a value-laden model which accepts a human being only in its perfection. As a consequence, he sees that the well-intentioned efforts to detect and eliminate genetic illness may result in society's determining a value for every member with a simplistic utilitarian yardstick. His warning is that the battle against genetic disorders has to be accompanied by respect for the autonomous decisions of the parents of the victims, and a societal commitment to provide comprehensive medical care to all patients afflicted by hereditary illness, malformations, and chromosomal abnormalities.

In the second chapter of this section, one particular clinical problem is selected for ethical analysis: the use of amniocentesis and the implementation of selective abortion. The different positions that have been presented in the literature are reviewed, and an approach is proposed that might be useful to the practicing pediatrician.

Daniel Callahan

1

THE MEANING AND SIGNIFICANCE OF GENETIC DISEASE: PHILOSOPHICAL PERSPECTIVES

I want to raise here the question of why we are concerned with genetic disease and how we might appropriately look upon it. I will leave to others a treatment of the various ethical problems which the detection and treatment of genetic disease pose. Instead, I will focus my attention on the kind of human, social, and cultural perspectives brought to bear on genetic disease, and the way in which they tend to establish the framework within which ethical issues are discerned and handled. This is important not only because these perspectives are interesting in themselves, but also because I am convinced that ethical systems, codes, and insights spring ultimately from assessments of the meaning and significance of human existence. All of us, I believe, have certain images of life, certain fundamental stances toward reality, certain sets of assumptions about the nature of things. Taken together, they help to determine the way questions are framed, priorities of interest established, emotional commitments made, fears, hopes, and anxieties aroused. The first question I want to pose concerning genetic disease is this: What image of human existence is pertinent as a framework for determining our response to the reality of genetic disease?

When I was about seven I was approached one day on a playground

Reprinted by courtesy of Hilton B et al: Ethical Issues in Human Genetics. New York, Plenum Publishing Co., 1973, pp 83–90.

by a very odd-looking boy of perhaps 12 or 13, stumbling, misshapen and with a rather silly, though friendly smile on his face. My reaction was a mixture of horror, fear, and curiosity. I wanted to stare at him and study him, but at the same time I wanted to run home as fast as I could. I resolved the dilemma at first by moving carefully backwards as he kept coming toward me, trying to keep him at a safe distance. But he kept coming and, eventually, I did run home, certain that if I did not he would "get me." He represented an alien, utterly inexplicable phenomenon.

No one, of course, had told me about Down's syndrome, and no one did for many years after. My parents said vaguely that he was "sick" and that "he wouldn't hurt me," but little more. That he was the child of a close neighbor, usually hidden, was something I had to deduce for myself. All the adults in the neighborhood, it seems, knew about him, but all tacitly engaged in a highly successful conspiracy to say nothing about the matter—indeed, to evade all pointed questions asked by innocent children. Eventually, the mongoloid I had encountered simply disappeared, no doubt into some institution.

I mention this incident because it seems to me to sum up one pervasive, almost instinctual human reaction to genetic disease. The defective human being has historically seemed a mysterious, awesome, terrifying creature—almost a separate, subhuman species—to be shunned altogether, explained away by means of elaborate religious mythologies, or given a special meaning, as an omen either of good or of evil. Of course, we now know more about genetic disease. We have some notion of why these hitherto strange creatures issue forth from the womb as defectives, and we think we have some ways of coping with what we are now able to classify as an abnormality.

But it would be a mistake to think that the old sense of mystery, awe, and terror does not live on. Surely the pervasive parental fear of bearing a defective child is not just because of the troubles of raising such a child, though that is a most serious matter. The fear seems much deeper than that, as if a defective child would represent a supreme undoing of the parents' image of themselves and reality. I am reminded of the conviction of many philosophers of antiquity that there is an irrational, irreducible absurd element in the universe, which constantly breaks through our visions and structures of ordered rationality. Genetic disease, long before it was labeled as that, was a case in point. One might in the instance of a hunting accident be able to discern a causal logic; the accident, however unacceptable, at least made sense. Genetic disease made no sense whatever; a defective child just arrived, out of some primeval darkness. A terror before the darkness still endures.

Yet, unlike our ancestors, we are no longer willing to be cowed. We are beginning to fight back, and the steps being taken follow a familiar script. We try to understand the mystery, by turning it into a problem rather than a mystery; then, with our cool-headed, rational explanation in hand we set ourselves to doing something about it—we label it a "disease" and then we try to "conquer" it. The change in our image of reality is evident here. Our ancestors had no choice but to be terrorized, and thus in compensation to find some symbolic means by which the philosophical absurdity of the defective existence could be understood and lived with. For our part, we act—fast, hard, and with all the technical means at our disposal.

The results are becoming evident. We are beginning to understand genetic disease, to know how to diagnose its presence, and, in some cases, how to cure it. Increasingly, it is becoming possible for those who do not want to bear defective children not to bear them. Since no one wants to bear such a child, just as they do not want to contract cancer or coronary disease, we are all that much the better off.

Yet at the level of broad philosophical perspective, I believe we should anticipate some problems. The conquest of genetic disease proceeds from the optimistic assumption that physical reality can be understood and that its aberrations can be minimized or eliminated. Nature can be brought to heel. That has been the assumption of the medical sciences generally, and its successes have served as the best possible arguments against those who still believe there is an absurd element in reality. Unfortunately, though, the fact of the matter is that we have just begun the conquest of genetic disease; it may be decades or centuries before the last defective child is born into the world. If a heuristic optimism is a necessity in order that the struggle against the disease is to go forward, this ought not to blind us to the fact that there is far more of what we do not know than of what we do, and far more genetic diseases that we have not conquered than we have.

In the meantime, during a great transition period that has no discernible end point, what ought to be the philosophical significance we attribute to genetic disease and genetically defective human beings? What ought our image of the world be and what place ought genetic disease to have within it? Let me point to some items on the present cultural horizon that seem to me to bespeak some dilemmas which need to be considered.

First, we still speak much of freedom of parental choice in the use of genetic information. And it is still common for genetic counselors to reassure parents that a defective fetus or child is "not their fault." Yet it is possible to detect tendencies which could eventually rob people of their choice and "blame" them for the defective children they bring into the world. If there is something of a paradox here at first sight, it soon disappears. For the corollary to giving people freedom of choice is to make them responsible for the choices they make. It is then only a very short step to begin distinguishing between responsible and irresponsible choices; social pressure begins to put in an appearance. Thus, while in principle the parents of a fetus with a detected case of Down's syndrome are still left free to decide whether to carry it to term, it is not difficult to discern an undercurrent in counseling literature and discussion that would classify such a decision as irresponsible. This is amplified in a subtle way. Abortion is said to be "medically indicated" in such cases, as if what is essentially an ethical decision has now become nothing but medical.

I am not concerned here with whether the decision in this or similar circumstances is irresponsible, or whether an abortion ought to be performed. I only want to point out that if and when we begin holding parents responsible for the children they bring into the world, and blaming them for what we take to be irresponsible choices, we may then have a result worse than that which flowed from the superstition of our ancestors. We will then share with our ancestors the view that a defective child is a curse but then, unlike them, provide no comfort whatever other than the ascetic reward of praise or blame for socially acceptable behavior in the face of the curse. In a word, it is simply not clear to me that in this circumstance an image of the world which, based on fierce rationality, would hold every person responsible for every jot and title of his or her behavior is altogether preferable to one which, while it could give them no choice, did not judge them either. And, of course, if we begin blaming those who make what we term "irresponsible" choices, then the freedom of choice now extolled in genetic counseling would become a mockery.

Second, while it has no doubt always been the case that parents of defective children have had to count the financial costs, the introduction of modern cost-accounting and cost-benefit analysis into the genetic equation adds a distinctively different element. We can now, quite literally, put a price on everyone's head, working out the long-term financial costs to individuals and societies of caring for a defective child.

But let us observe a curiosity. It was counted a great advance of the modern mind when a bookkeeping God, with his minutely maintained ledger of good and bad deeds, was noisily rejected. Yet here we are, beginning to keep our own books, and using them increasingly as a determinant in deciding whether or not defectives should be allowed the privilege of birth, and their parents the privilege of parenthood. Moreover, we seem to have forgotten the reason why the bookkeeping God was rejected—because it seemed eminently unjust, insensitive, and outrageous that a scorecard be kept on human lives. Indeed, we are even worse than that old God; for at least in his ledger everything was supposedly recorded. But our cost-benefit analysis totes up one item only—what the financial liability of the defective will be, what he will cost us in terms of taxes, institutional facilities, the time of medical personnel, and so on. Needless to say, this kind of reckoning is prone to be weak in comparing the costs of the defective against the cost of other patently foolish public and private expenditures which are accepted with barely a word of protest. What is society spending on cosmetics this year? Nor does this kind of reckoning have much to say about ways of reconstructing the social and political order to make possible a more humane treatment of those considered a social liability—the poor, the aged, the unfit. No, for the kind of cost-benefit analysis which seems to be emerging in genetic calculations goes only in the cost direction; it is seemingly assumed that the benefits to a society which decided simply to bear the costs of humane care are either nonexistent or simply too intangible to be worth much bother.

Third, behind the human horror at genetic defectiveness lurks, one must suppose, an image of the perfect human being. The very language of "defect," "abnormality," "disease," and "risk" presupposes such an image, a kind of prototype of perfection. In the past there seemed little which could be done to realize the prototype; it was contemplated as a platonic form, well out of reach. Eventually, a kind of wisdom developed. Since it appeared clear that even if there is a perfect human being to be conceived or imagined, the price of pursuing and imposing it is very high in terms of the ways it can change our response to actually existing human beings. Human diversity began to be appreciated and justified. In fact, behind modern society's at least verbal commitment to civil rights, to justice for all, lies a rejection of images of individual perfection and uniformity. A similar pattern has been manifest in even the purely scientific sphere, with a rejection in biology and zoology of monotypical modes of analysis and classification (which stressed a fixed, static concept of type) in favor of a populationist approach (which makes room for a richer appreciation of individual variation).

Yet because of the advances in the detection and cure of genetic disease—the ghost of the perfect human being, once sensibly laid to rest, is putting in his appearance again. And I believe we are beginning to see evidence of what this means: a heightened anxiety on the part of prospective parents about bearing a defective child, increased social pressure against those who would bear a child deviating from the norm of perfection, and, at what I hope is not the leading edge but a fringe only, hints that the sensible society of the future will of course deny parents the right to bring into the world any child who could not measure up, who would be a burden upon society.

There have surely been abuses and a good deal of plain silliness in recent rejections of purported ethical absolutes and ethical objectivity, of fixed codes, of rigid notions of the "human" and the "nonhuman," of the worthy and the unworthy, of static notions of perfection and imperfection. But on the whole, this rejection has helped to soften life, to provide a defense against the totalitarian reformer, to widen our appreciation of the value of human differences, variations, and dissimilarities, to lead us to construct visions of political and social orders which can encompass and profit from variety. An image of man based on a pluralistic rather than a monistic conception of reality has been hard-won. It would be a supreme irony if, in the name of even greater progress, there was reintroduced the old monistic, monotypical kind of thinking, this time, as before, in the name of value, good order, and a mythical notion of perfection.

Fourth, every image of the world and reality carries with it a correlative view of the nature of human community. It is not for nothing that political reformers and revolutionaries (think only of Karl Marx) have felt that the condition for a change in ethical and political thinking is, first of all, a change in metaphysical thinking. An egalitarian social structure can, only with difficulty and patch-work logic, be built upon a metaphysic of fixed hierarchical realities. Participatory democracy has nothing going for it in a society that secretly believes that some people are inherently lower than others and thus not fit to govern themselves.

It would be a mistake to say that past human societies adapted happily and well to the reality of genetic disease and defect. Yet there did develop the humane response that society as a whole should share the burden of caring for the defective, that the parents or family should not be left with sole responsibility for the care and survival of the defective. Moreover, in laws against infanticide, child neglect, and abuse, there was reflected a belief that society has an obligation toward children, an obligation which holds good regardless of their physical or mental condition. We can see in these historical developments a concept of community and society which tried to respond to human diversity, even that diversity represented by the grossly abnormal. So, too, it was perceived that any effective recognition of diversity—which means a recognition of actual inequalities of individual assets and liabilities in society—required a joint sharing of responsibility by all for all, so that those least equipped by nature or nurture to function would not be inevitable losers.

This cultural development represented a great milestone in human history, even if our society and most others have hardly succeeded in living up to the obligations which it entailed. We created public institutions for defectives, only too often to treat them like animals once we gave them the benefit of admission to those institutions. Nonetheless, the introduction of the very notion of common and public responsibility represented a triumph of great magnitude. A triumph, I am sorry to say, which would all be for nothing if we accept the idea that defectives and their parents have no right to burden the rest of us with their troubles, or that it is naive to find a social solution for a problem which can be done away with by a scientific solution.

I would not want to be misunderstood here. Nothing I have said should be construed as an objection to the further development and refinement of genetic knowledge and the art of genetic counseling. On the contrary, the suffering brought on by genetic disease warrants nothing less than a full-scale social, scientific, and economic effort to eliminate, cure, or alleviate these afflictions. My concern, rather, is with the spirit in which such an effort is undertaken, with the kind of philosophical perspective which should lie behind it, and with the social context in which it is carried out.

Genetic disease will not be done away with overnight, if ever. At the simplest level, there is at least a requirement that people's hopes not be raised too high too precipitately; that will just set the stage for even more suffering. More important though is the question of how we are to continue living in the company of genetic disease, even as vigorous steps are taken to minimize its impact. As Professor Crow has emphasized, the reality of genetic disease is that it is a recurrent disease brought about by the continued reintroduction of defective genes by mutation. The overarching dilemma I have tried to sketch comes to this: How can we manage both to live humanely with genetic disease and yet to conquer it at the same time? Both goals seem imperative and yet the logic of each is different. We cure disease by ceasing to romanticize it, by gathering our powers to attack it, by making it an enemy to be conquered. We learn to live with a disease, however, in a very difficult way; by trying to accept and cherish those who manifest the disease, by shaping social structures and institutions which will soften the individual suffering brought on by the disease, by refusing to make the bearer of the disease our economic, social, or political enemy.

Our communal task, I believe, is to find a way of combining both logics. That will not be easy, if only because most people find it easier to cope with one idea than with two at the same time. It will mean, for instance, simultaneously working to improve the societal treatment and respect accorded those born with defects, and working to extend our genetic knowledge and applying it to genetic counseling. It will mean taking the idea of free choice seriously, allowing parents to make their own choice without penalizing them socially for the choices they make, or condemning them for those choices which will increase the financial costs to society. Part of the very meaning of human community, I would contend, entails a willingness of society to bear the social costs of individual freedom.

It will mean some care in the way we use language. As physical organisms we stand "at risk" of genetic disease, as do our children and our descendants; as cultural beings, however, we stand "at risk" also in another sense, of seeing our values, our better instincts, and our humanity diseased and crippled. If odds are to be calculated, then let both sets of risks be included in our general equation. Moreover, if the "risk" of genetic disease is to be calculated, and better calculated, let it be remembered that no set of mathematical statistics can, by themselves, "indicate" what we ought to do in response to the realities they delineate. That requires the introduction of ethical premises, and those premises, in turn, require some coherent notion of what the human good is. When we speak of the good of "the patient," let it not be the case, in the first place, that we use the term "patient" only for those we think desirable to treat (using some clinical term for the rest—fetus, conceptus, neonate); or, in the second place, that the decision if and how to treat a patient not be made a matter of how we, as individuals or community, happen to feel about the intrinsic worth of that patient. Beyond that, particular care is needed when we speak of someone or some group's "good." It is not all that easy to know what is good for the individual, for the family, and for society, though one might gather otherwise in light of the many confident statements made on the subject. As a descriptive term indicating deviation from a statistical mean, the word "abnormal" can be very helpful; as a philosophical term, indicating some mandatory level of social and genetic fitness—a prototype of human perfection—it can be very hazardous.

To conquer a disease is to reflect a view of the world. It is also to create a partially new world and a new view of human possibilities. How we go about dealing with genetic disease—the kinds of counseling techniques developed, the professional consensuses which emerge, the attitudes developed toward carriers of defects and toward the children many of them will bear, the kinds of choices which emerge and the positions taken on the nature of those choices—will both reflect one world and bring another into being. That is a heavy burden to bear, and we had better be aware of it.

Tomas J. Silber, M.D.

2

AMNIOCENTESIS AND SELECTIVE ABORTION

Each new power won by man
is a power over man as well
—C. S. Lewis

The purpose of this chapter is to present a bioethical inquiry into the moral problems posed by the screening and abortion of the defective fetus.[1] It is now possible to detect numerous genetic defects before birth. The technology to do this is no longer experimental nor reduced to a few medical centers and specialists. On the contrary, such technology has been standardized and incorporated into our medical armamentarium. Nieswander's Manual of Obstetric Diagnosis and Therapy, a widely read text, lists the following as the acceptable practice in our profession.[2]

> Amniocentesis is accomplished by inserting a needle into the amniotic cavity, usually with ultrasound control, to withdraw fluid. The fluid can be used for diagnostic tests directly, or it can be centrifuged and incubated to grow the embryonic cells it contains for chromosome analysis. This procedure is usually performed at about 16 weeks from the last menstrual period. Before that time, there is insufficient fluid (or cells in the fluid), and later, insufficient time will elapse between the harvest of the cells (three to five weeks) and the 20-week gestational interval most desirable for an indicated abortion.

Many students are now graduating from medical school for whom these practices are as natural as the use of immunizations has been for most of us practicing pediatricians. The problem that this presents is that each time

Reprinted by courtesy of Pediatric Annals 10:31, 1981.

that a technique is made part of our professional culture it becomes very easy to lose our perspective on the ethical issues involved in its use. This is poignantly expressed when one questions if what *can* be done *ought* to be done.

Ethical issues related to amniocentesis per se are often ignored by physicians and laymen alike, probably because they are overshadowed by the more central issue of abortion. Nevertheless, amniocentesis presents its own problems. When the procedure first became available it captured the imagination of some ethicists who opposed amniocentesis because no informed consent can be obtained from a fetus. This argument is still presented forcefully by Ramsey, who works under the assumption that the fetus has a moral status.[3] The opposition to this view comes mainly from those who do not accept Ramsey's basic assumption, and interestingly, also from those who claim that fetuses have a "right to be born normal" or even a "right not to be born."

Another important ethical question raised by amniocentesis is whether or not commitment to an abortion should be a prerequisite to the realization of the procedure. This position was the prevailing practice in many centers in the late 60s and early 70s and was based on the view that one should try to avoid a useless waste of medical resources and also try to minimize unnecessary risks to the fetus. This policy is still practiced in some areas with the rationale that though the fetal morbidity and mortality from amniocentesis is low, it is still sufficient to warrant the contraindication of the procedure in those instances where there is no prospect of a therapeutic application. Veatch opposed this view persuasively: "Even when no medical use (other than abortion) can be made of the prenatal diagnosis, it seems that some might opt for amniocentesis and make use of the intervening days to make what they may consider to be a weighty and moral decision about abortion."[4] I also argue against the withholding position, basing my judgment on the fact that important psychological needs, such as the necessity for anticipatory guidance, may be overlooked when solely an "organic" approach is considered.

The majority of those who oppose amniocentesis do so because they view it as an immediate link to abortion. Thomas Szasz once suggested that abortion relates to medical judgment exactly as capital punishment relates to electrical engineering, and indeed medical knowledge is not sufficient preparation for the abortion debate. Ethical reflection on abortion has been acquiring particular sophistication over the last 20 years, and it is not possible to do justice to this body of knowledge in a single chapter.[5] Nevertheless, I propose that the following four points may synthesize, for the purpose of this article, the divergent ethical beliefs that recur most often in the abortion debate:

1. Abortion is the equivalent of infanticide. Hence the whole procedure is morally wrong (Ramsey,[3] Noonan[6]).

2. The fetus is not a person and has no moral claims; abortion presents no moral problems (Tooley,[7] Englehart[8]).

3. Personhood is conferred neither at conception nor at birth, but it is a developmental process extending over a period of time. An abortion following amniocentesis is therefore a very serious decision because such an abortion is of necessity a late one (Brody,[9] Fletcher[10]).

4. The fetus has a moral claim to development and birth but not an absolute claim against all other considerations (Thomson,[11] Silber[12]).

The ethical debate about abortions following a diagnosis of fetal illness or fetal malformation is *not* identical to the ethical debate about abortion in general and deserves a separate analysis. As a matter of fact, this type of abortion has received its own name: selective abortion. There are few grounds for abortion stronger than a serious genetic defect. Yet, two positions clearly emerge in relationship to this issue. One position "builds up" and favors the abortion of defective fetuses and insists on providing safeguards against indiscriminate abortion (for example, through quality counseling). The other position "builds down," arguing that selective abortion is morally wrong and permissible, if at all, only in special cases of tremendous gravity.

The fact that a child could be born defective is not seen as a sufficient reason for abortion. Lebacqz best summarizes arguments of the adversaries of selective abortion, stating that abortion violates the principle of justice and threatens the traditional life-preserving orientation of medicine.[13] Lebacqz develops the theme that in a situation of conflict, priority ought to be given to the weaker party. In this instance, to overrule the unequal position of the fetus would be to ignore the principle of equality. She thus concludes that the only ethical valid course of action is the maintenance of a fetus, even if defective, and she urges the medical profession to abandon the practice of selective abortion.

This argument has been answered as follows: justice does not require equality, it does require that men share one another's fate (Rawls). (It has even been postulated that justice requires sharing the genetic load of mankind—and, therefore, the duty of reducing its total burden.) Finally, Lebacqz' opponents bring up the principle of beneficence in order to outweigh her arguments: entire families are being protected from the emotional and financial strain of bearing and rearing a defective child and therefore selective abortion may be justified on a consequential ground. This challenge to Lebacqz pushes for another interpretation of selective abortion; rather than describing the procedure as resulting in the death of the patient (the fetus) it views it as a case of disease prevention. Hare's idea comes to mind here; we are urged to value the benefit to future potential persons, such as the child that will be born in the future in place of the defective fetus aborted in the present.[14]

Partisans of selective abortion agree on the basis of the principle of beneficence. But other complex problems remain. How serious must a defect be to warrant abortion? What should be the attitude toward abortion in cases where remedial treatment would be available to the child who would be born defective? What about the healthy fetuses that are aborted when x-linked diseases are being considered? Where do you draw the line?

Pediatricians share even another worry: what is the effect on parents of being in the position of having to make this decision? Addressing this concern, Fletcher perceptively comments: "Even if the diagnosis given by genetic investigation was negative you have nonetheless (at least) entertained the idea of the death of your baby. To contemplate the death of your baby in the third month of pregnancy changes very seriously the attitude we, as a society, usually have toward our babies."[10] Others have speculated that selective abortion might subtly worsen the attitude of our society toward defective persons. Kass warns us: "A child with a genetic defect, born at the time when most of his potential fellow sufferers were destroyed prenatally, is liable to be looked on by the community as one unfit to be alive, as a second class human type. He may be seen as a person who needs not to have been and who would not have been if someone had gotten to him in time."[15] This is a serious example of the "slippery slope" argument. Moreover, the existence of defective persons can never be prevented, since in addition to genetic disorders, other processes such as birth injury, accidents, abuse, and disease all leave their toll. If all defective people ever get lumped into one inferior class, this would have a disastrous influence on our whole concept of what is meant to be human.

Paradoxically, some oppose widespread selective abortion on genetic grounds: many of the transmitted genetic conditions for which abortion is being sought are treatable: but, more to the point, when carrier parents opt for an abortion, they are encouraged to have more children and therefore the net result could be an increase in defective genes in the population. In addition, a tendency may grow to reduce efforts in research and therapeutic innovation for those conditions that may come to be considered remediable through selective abortion.

Where does all this leave us in our role as pediatricians? Although involved in societal concerns, our immediate obligation is to serve individual patients and families. Particular individuals will ask us about amniocentesis and selective abortion. I, like many, had the opportunity to think about this on numerous opportunities, and I still find myself reflecting about two somewhat contradictory experiences. On one hand, I feel an inherent repugnance to fetal destruction, stemming perhaps from my years of caring for the fetus' "closest relative," the newborn premature baby. Having participated in bitter team fights for the lives of many "little ones," I can see an awful paradox in the termination of fetal development. In other words, I sense I have a particular relationship with a future human being. I recognize him/her as part of my species. More specifically, in my identity as a pediatrician I experience emotionally my loyalty to the fetus.

On the other hand, on reviewing my almost 20 years of medical practice, I recall seeing families devastated by the slow dying of patients with Tay-Sachs disease, seeing children with serious neurologic ailments draining their families' resources for years, seeing children with severe deformities being left to vegetate in less-than-acceptable institutions, seeing serious emotional disturbances in the often neglected siblings of defective children, seeing the fate of inhumanely abused retarded patients, and, grieving over all this, I cannot help but often think: could not all this have been avoided?

Yes, the ethical response to the abortion of the defective or the possibly defective fetus is complex, and consensus may be difficult to reach. Nevertheless, I propose to conclude this chapter with ten propositions for the practicing pediatrician in the hope of generating further thoughts and contributions:

1. Every pediatrician has a duty to keep up-to-date with the current development of prenatal and postnatal screening and, when appropriate, to share this knowledge with his patients.
2. The decision to undergo amniocentesis does not need to be related to the decision to undergo an abortion, but patients need to be informed accurately about the risks involved in the procedure. Amniocentesis is a sophisticated medical procedure and should not be used unless a physician agrees that it is indicated.
3. Most of the women who undergo amniocentesis for prenatal diagnosis are relieved of their anxieties. Still, the physician needs to inform parents realistically that a negative amniocentesis cannot be construed as a guarantee for normality.
4. In those cases in which amniocentesis is positive, the pediatrician is obliged to share with the family his knowledge of the outcome of the feared condition as well as the current societal resources to help the potential victim.
5. It is not the pediatrician's role to recommend a particular decision, though he might share his moral and ethical convictions whenever he is genuinely asked for an opinion. It is fundamental, though, that the physician's personal view not be forced upon his patients.
6. Likewise, from a procedural standpoint, it is not appropriate for physicians to establish lists of genetic disorders in which termination of pregnancy is indicated. Ethical reflections should not be replaced by technical expertise.
7. Once the parents have reached their decision, the physician's support is needed and is extremely important.
8. All pediatricians should be alert to the fact that the timing of selective abortion coincides with the time the fetal movements have been felt, and thus this might predispose the mother to depression, to the mourning of her loss.
9. Our attention as clinicians and as researchers should be directed to learning how selective abortion affects both parents as well as other children in the family.
10. Finally, the pediatrician has an important role in giving medical and psychologic support to the survivors of conditions that may have been eliminated through abortion, and who at times may now come to see themselves as "superfluous" or "a burden." The pediatrician has an important responsibility, shared with the rest of the community, to ensure that all handicapped children and their families be provided with adequate resources.

REFERENCES

1. Birch C, Abrecht P: Genetics and the Quality of Life. Elmsford. NY, Pergamon Press 1975.
2. Neiswander KR: Manual of Obstetrics, Diagnosis and Therapy. Boston, Little Brown and Company. 1980
3. Ramsey P: Screening: an ethicist's view. *In* Hilton B et al. (eds.): Ethical Issues in Human Genetics. New York, Plenum Press. 1973.
4. Veatch R: Ethical issues in genetics. *In* Veatch R: Progress in Medical Genetics 10:223–264, 1974.
5. Callahan D: Abortion: Choice and Morality. New York, Macmillan Company, 1970.
6. Noonan JT Jr:An almost absolute value in history. *In* Noonan JT Jr (ed.): The Morality of Abortion: Legal and Historical Perspectives. Cambridge. Mass, Harvard University Press. 1970.
7. Tooley M: Abortion and infanticide. Phil. Publ. Affairs 2:37–65, 1972.
8. Englehardt HT: The ontology of abortion. Ethics 84:217–234, 1974.
9. Brody B: On the humanity of the fetus. *In* Perkins RI (ed.): Abortion: Pro and Con. Cambridge. Mass, Schenkman Publishing Company, 1974.
10. Fletcher J: The brink: The parent-child bond in the genetic revolution. Theological Studies 33:457–485, 1972.
11. Thomson JJ: In defense of abortion. Philos Publ Affairs 1:47–66, 1971.
12. Silber TJ: Abortion in adolescents: Ethical dimension. Adolescence 15:461–474, 1980.
13. Lebacqz KA: Prenatal diagnosis and selective abortion. Linacre Q 40:109–127, 1973.
14. Hare RM: Survival of the weakest. *In* Gorovitz S (ed.): Moral Problems in Medicine. Englewood Cliffs, NJ, Prentice Hall. 1976.
15. Kass LR: The new biology: What price reliving man's estate? Science (November 19, 1971), 779–788.

SECTION ONE FURTHER READINGS

1. Beauchamp TL, Childress JT: Principles of Biomedical Ethics. New York, Oxford University Press, 1979.
2. Brody H: Ethical Decisions in Medicine, 2nd Ed. Boston, Little, Brown, & Co., 1981.
3. Englehardt HT: Bioethics in Pluralist Societies. Persp Biol Med 26:64–78, 1982.
4. Fletcher J: Indicators of Humanhood. Hastings Center Report 2:1, 1972.
5. Ramsey P: Ethics at the Edges of Life. New Haven, Yale University Press, 1978.
6. Reich WT: Encyclopedia of Bioethics. New York, The Free Press, 1978.

SECTION TWO

LIFE AND DEATH

Any discussion of life and death raises moral issues. A parallel exists between the concerns relating to selective abortion of genetically defective fetuses (Chapter 1) and the practice of letting defective newborns die. William Silverman makes a case for accepting the decision made by parents of defective newborns to refuse medical intervention that could otherwise be life saving. He does this on straightforward consequential grounds. Thus, when a deformed newborn's life only offers the prospect of suffering and deterioration, family upheaval, and disintegration, the course of nontreatment is seen as the most merciful and right thing to do. This argument is rejected in Norman Fost's view; he feels the obligation to act with the best interest of the child in mind. This, he insists, may conflict with that of the parent, especially if in all truth, one cannot ascertain whether a limited life is to be preferred to no life at all.

Decision-making becomes even more painful when the agreement to withhold care is allowed to be made in response to an adolescent's request, as is illustrated by John Schowalter's article. In the closing chapter of this section, Silber addresses the moral dilemma confronting the adolescent who is considering abortion.

William A. Silverman, M.D.

3

MISMATCHED ATTITUDES ABOUT NEONATAL DEATH

Extravagance is a notable characteristic of human reproduction, as it is in all animal species: the majority of offspring launched at conception die before or soon after birth. For example, it is estimated that 40% of human pregnancies end in spontaneous miscarriage; a little more than half of these occur so early that a woman may not even realize she is pregnant.[1] (Major chromosomal abnormalities are a leading cause of this substantial toll in fetal life.) Many unwanted pregnancies are intentionally terminated (approximately 30% of pregnant women in the United States chose abortions during 1979[2]); and an unknown number of liveborn infants are neglected, abandoned, or killed before they reach the age of one month.

These biologic imperfections and what seem to be defects in parenting behavior are not new. What is novel, over the few million-or-so years of human existence, is the idea that succor of *all* viable babies is a desirable social goal. The history of efforts to accomplish this ideal has been marked by continuous conflict because the attitudes of parents have not always been congruent with the views of authorities. A recurring question has been, Whose baby is it, anyway?[3]

For countless millennia, despite differing cultural contexts, parental at-

Reprinted with permission of The Hastings Center, Institute of Society, Ethics, and the Life Sciences, 360 Broadway, Hastings-on-Hudson, NY 10706.

titudes, as manifested by overt behavior, have been fairly consistent. On the whole, parents have acted on the assumption that each baby is a personal possession and that they are the ones to decide whether to invest the economic and psychologic resources needed for the transformation of their completely dependent biologic creation into an independent social being. However, they have not gone unchallenged. Over the centuries, three Western institutions have in turn taken the lead to develop social policy aimed at limiting parental autonomy with respect to offspring: the first was religion; the second, law; and for the last hundred years, medicine has taken on the task. The opportunities for a mismatch between the attitudes of parents and of authorities have grown out of these historic movements, as the following brief survey will show.

RELIGIOUS AND LEGAL PROSCRIPTIONS AGAINST INFANTICIDE

Infanticide is the oldest method of human family planning. Our prehistoric ancestors abandoned or killed neonates (especially females) to balance reproductive pressures in relation to means of subsistence.[4] Organized religion, beginning with the ancient Hebrews, made the first efforts to take these planning decisions out of parental hands.[5] Prior to the time of Abraham, the distinction between the value of children and of animals was blurred. But when Abraham substituted a ram as a burnt offering to God in place of his son Isaac, a clear line was drawn by the leaders of the new faith. Still, some parents in ancient Israel continued to practice infanticide: as late as the time of Isaiah they were criticized for the habit of "slaying the children in the valleys under the clefts of the rocks."[6] The proscription against infanticide was apparently meant to apply to infants more than a month old: in early Jewish law (especially the Pharisaic Code) a child less than that age was not a legal person, and death was often considered an abortion.[7] The father alone had the absolute power of life and death over members of his family, including the right to decide the fate of newborn babies.[8] Postneonatal infanticide probably declined in part because the biblical injunction "Be fruitful and multiply" was an important commandment with respect to military strength; Abraham was promised: ". . . your descendants shall capture the gates of their enemies."

Justinian notes the Roman law (*Lex pompeia de parricidiis,* passed under the consulship of Pompeius in 52 B.C.) that provided an awesome punishment for anyone who hastened the death of a relative.

> He will be punished, not by the sword, nor by fire, nor by an ordinary mode of punishment, but he will be sewed up in a sack with a dog, a cock, a viper, and an ape, and enclosed in this horrible prison he is to be, according to the nature of the place, thrown into the sea, or into the river . . . .[9]

Interestingly, the term *parricidium* included the murder of a child who was killed by the mother or grandfather, but not by the father.

With the coming of Christianity, there was a specific theologic motivation for the importance of species membership: the belief that all born of human parents were immortal and destined for an eternity of bliss or everlasting torment.[10] Early Christian leaders thundered against infanticide as a heathen practice: they insisted that all human life be held inviolable (although the exact fetal age at which ensoulment and thus "true human-ness" was considered to take place was a matter of shifting doctrine). However, the proscriptive attitude of the early Christian emperors was not universally held.[11] Constantine never explicitly forbade infanticide and later emperors did nothing to abolish exposure of infants or the sale of children as slaves. It was not until 529 A.D. (under the Justinian Code) that the subjection of foundlings to slavery was prohibited. But the Fourth Table of the Code referred to the father of the family who was *bidden* to destroy deformed children, and the absolute power of the head of the house over the life of his children was affirmed.[12]

There is general agreement that the disparity between religious and legal proclamations and parental practice continued. Child murder was common, even in the most developed Western countries, but a distinction grew up between active and passive measures. In the early Middle Ages, infanticide was punishable by law, exposure was not. And abandonment "was practiced on a gigantic scale with absolute impunity, noticed by writers with most frigid indifference and, at least in the case of destitute parents, considered a very venial [easily pardonable] offense."[13]

The penalty for premeditated infanticide by violent means was severe in the Middle Ages. Nuremberg court and prison records indicate that prior to 1500, women convicted of the crime—principally unmarried girls—were buried alive, often with gruesome refinements.[14] During the sixteenth century, the usual method was drowning, and after 1580, decapitation. But the charge of deliberate murder was difficult to prove. Accidental "overlaying" in the parents' bed or suffocation by bedclothes did occur, but how could one prove intent to kill? Still, because large numbers of babies were involved, the suspicion of intentional infanticide could not be dispelled. The authorities contented themselves with imposing a penance: in the case of married women, to live for at least a year on bread and water.

During the eighteenth century in France, Germany, and a number of other European countries, the punishment for abandoning or killing a baby was usually a cruel death by a variety of means, the most merciful of which was decapitation. Other methods echoed the Roman and medieval punishments—burial alive, impalement, and "sacking." Maria W. Piers describes a scene in which an infanticidal mother was stuffed into a black sack together with a dog, a cat, a rooster, and a viper, just as the Roman law had dictated. The sack was submerged in water for six hours, as choir boys sang *Aus tiefer Noth schrei ich zu Dir* ("Out of the depths I cry to thee," from Psalm 129, "De Profundis"). Then the deceased was interred.[15]

Despite the inevitable difficulty of interpreting scattered and perhaps incomplete historical evidence, it is clear that large numbers of women, faced with the opposing demands of a harsh reality and the idealized values of church and state, continued to risk barbaric punishments by committing offensive acts in what appears (from this distance) to have been attempts to control their own lives. Although parents who could afford it sometimes showed a striking degree of concern over neonatal mortality, infanticide persisted despite all denunciations by the church and all the penalties of the law.[16]

Through the centuries, sporadic efforts were made to deal with the problem of unwanted babies in a nonpunitive way by housing them in small foundling homes, but it was not until the eighteenth century that religious and philanthropic institutions attempted to rescue infants on a large scale in asylums and foundling hospitals. However, this merely changed the time and the site of child deaths. The efforts were dubbed "legalized infanticide."

In mid-nineteenth century England, an observer commented on what appeared to be "great indifference displayed by parents . . ." with regard to infant life.[17] While evidence of numbers of infants affected is not available, women employed in factories and fields placed their babies with "killer nurses" (also called "angel makers"): the caretakers made short shrift of their charges with generous doses of Godfrey's Cordial (a concoction of opium, treacle, and sassafras). The practice was institutionalized and became known as "baby farming." Some women paid a small premium (£ 1) to enroll their infants in burial clubs. After a decent interval, the children died of starvation, neglect, or poisoning; and the mothers collected £ 3 to £ 5 in benefits. Some women joined ten or more clubs, reaping rich returns from the schemes. A survey of the British press in the 1860s revealed frequent reports of dead infants found under bridges, in parks, in culverts and ditches, and in cesspools.[18] Infanticide in England during this period became the subject of much official agitation, which led to the first Infant Life Protection Act in 1872.

English juries, however, were reluctant to convict mothers for the murder of their newborn infants. They would grasp at any suggestion that the baby had been stillborn, died in the course of childbirth, or had been accidentally killed.[19] Infanticide was often excused on the basis of temporary insanity ("puerperal psychosis" and "lactational insanity" became common terms). A Capital Commission of 1864–1866 noted that it was "established practice" in the British Home Office to advise commutation of the death penalty when a woman was convicted of murdering her own child while it was less than, or not more than, twelve months. One witness at the hearings was bold enough to hint that less harm was done in neonatal homicides than in other cases: "You cannot estimate the loss to the child itself, you know nothing about it at all. With regard to the public it causes no alarm, because it is a crime which can be committed only by mothers upon their newly born children."

There is evidence that a less punitive attitude toward the crime of infanticide extended into the modern era. For example, in 1936 arguments were advanced to modify English legislation so that it would correspond more closely with public feeling and with the widespread use of the prerogative of mercy by the courts. It was proposed that a mother who killed her "infant"—up to the age of eight years—would be exempted from the death penalty: the proposal would have widened the definition of the mother's confused state of mind to include "distress and despair arising from the solicitude for her child or extreme poverty or other causes." Although this provision was not enacted, it indicated that the conflicts concerning this disturbing problem were not yet resolved. Centuries of effort had been unsuccessful in obliterating the ancient view that distinguished between the death of a neonate and the loss of life of a self-conscious, rational human being.

In reviewing the evolution of infanticide laws in England and the status of the infant's life in American law (which makes no distinction between homicide and infanticide), one researcher found evidence that in practice under both systems the infant does, indeed, have lower status than the adult. The researcher concluded that "such status does not represent an erosion of ethical or religious values nor is it evidence of a brutal society, but rather demonstrates society's continued ambivalence toward the inherent sanctity of life and realistic judgment on the quality of life."[20]

Embedded in the distinction between newborn infants and adults, for example, is the difference between abstract and concrete rights.[21] Whereas abstract rights, such as justice and the right to survive, are considered to belong to every person, concrete rights take into account the possibility of a conflict of claims: the projected needs of a biologically dependent sentient being—who is not yet rational or self-conscious—competing with demands of others in the family who are in full possession of all the characteristics of personhood.[22] Those living under miserable conditions have often been unwilling to grant full personhood to all their offspring solely for the purpose of fulfilling the moral expectations of theologians and legislators.

THE RISE OF MEDICAL INFLUENCE

About the time that other institutions were moving away from absolutist approaches to the complicated social problem, some physicians began to take an active role in preventing women from terminating their unwanted pregnancies or doing away with their offspring. An English physician, William B. Ryan, wrote in 1846, "We cannot ignore the fact that the crime of infanticide, as well as that of criminal abortion, is widespread and on the increase."[23] He and another doctor, John Curgeven, led a delegation of medical men who called on the government to check the practice of child murder. Curgeven founded the Infant Protection Society that pressed for passage of the 1872 Act to protect infant lives. In the United States, Dr. Horatio Robinson Storer and members of the newly formed American Medical Association—not ecclesiastic authorities—mounted a campaign (beginning in 1847) that led to the passage of antiabortion laws in all of the states.[24] Dr. E.P. Christian stated the high aims of the lobbying movement: "It is not sufficient that the medical profession should set up a standard of morality for themselves, but the people are to be educated up to it."

Organized efforts to save less-than-robust newborn infants began in France a century ago.[25] Following the immense loss of life from military action and the months of famine in the Franco-Prussian War (1870–71), "feeble" neonates began to receive more attention from obstetricians and nurses. Ingenious incubators *(couveuses)* and tube-feeding techniques (French *gavage*) were developed to prevent what were previously regarded as "expected losses" of infant life. In England, the steady fall of the birthrate, beginning in 1871, was cited by physicians at the turn of the century as evidence for the need to use the new French methods to conserve the lives of all infants "even the prematurely born . . . for economic as well as sentimental reasons."[26]

Early on, it was found that when groups of "weaklings"—especially the prematurely born—were reared in specialized nurseries, recurrent waves of infection quickly snuffed out the lives of the small patients.[27] To lower this risk, precautions were taken to isolate the susceptible babies in glass-enclosed hospital units. In the sterile surroundings, highly skilled and carefully scrubbed nurses cared for their charges; they took elaborate measures to prevent the introduction of infections, and, significantly, they forbade parents to come into physical contact with their fragile new offspring.

The rigid guidelines for the care of small infants slowly spread throughout the Western world, sometimes under very curious circumstances. Beginning in 1896, live premature infants were exhibited at expositions in many countries to demonstrate "the new scientific methods of care."[28] The bizarre Incubator Baby Exhibits at fairs, and later in amusement areas like Coney Island, were tacitly sanctioned by a curious public who paid to see the shows. Parents of the neonates also seemed to accept this peculiar arrangement; indeed, they were often too accepting, for many quickly lost interest in their children, and there was some difficulty in convincing them to assume parental responsibilities when the time came to send the fattened babies home.

The incubator-baby sideshows faded from the scene after the 1939 Worlds Fair in New York, about the time premature infant nurseries began to proliferate in large hospitals throughout the United States. These specialized care facilities operated according to the sideshow model: strict isolation measures discouraged traffic in the units, parents had to observe their babies from a distance through glass, and even physicians were discouraged from touching their patients too frequently.[29]

I became interested in the problems of premature infants during this era in 1944, and I quickly became aware of the agony of parents at the birth of a very small or malformed infant. Although most parents expressed concern for the immediate prospects of life, ambivalent attitudes were the rule. Frequently fathers and mothers begged me not to "try too hard" to keep their children alive. In the early years, there were few effective techniques to prevent the early deaths, and the fate of the tiny babies after the first few days was not in my hands but in those of skilled nurses. The nurses quickly became attached to the small survivors, while parents were passive observers. The phenomenon of parental detachment, first noted in the incubator-baby sideshows, was repeated many times in the premature infant nurseries.

As the life-support techniques for newborn infants became more effective in the 1960s, the premature nurseries changed radically. Not only were many previously nonviable small infants kept alive, but parents were encouraged to enter the new neonatal intensive care units (NICUs) and to establish a physical and emotional bond with the new baby. Most parents entered this frightening environment with apprehension, but many quickly overcame their fears with the support of empathetic nurses and physicians. I observed, however, that some parents were unable to overcome their ambivalent feelings at the birth of a very small or otherwise less-than-perfect baby. The smaller the infant and the more serious the imperfection, the more common were the mixed feelings about survival. I was painfully aware that parental reactions were strongly influenced by my words and those of the nurses, and that nonverbal communication—not only from caretakers but from the impressive physical setting and the awesome life-support machinery—played a significant role in determining how the parents expressed their feelings about this crisis in their lives. Since then, the technology has grown rapidly, and with it even more opportunities for conflict and for misreading attitudes about neonatal death.

A 1979 news item illustrates the kind of difficulty that may arise on the modern scene.[30] In describing Mignon, born seventeen weeks before term and weighing 482 grams, the reporter quotes her physicians:

> She has been plagued with frequent kidney failures, liver problems that defy textbook definition, and the usual lung problems . . . at seven months after delivery she is hanging in there. We have kept the [umbilical artery] catheter in her aorta all the way, so her hyperalimentation has been intra-arterial . . . she can't suck because of the endotracheal tube . . . of course, she has been constantly on PEEP . . . But with no spontaneous breathing, all mechanical ventilation, her lungs are pretty damaged now . . .[30]

I find it disturbing that the reporter made no mention of Mignon's parents. What was their opinion of this impressive flexing of hardware?

In another article, this one written by the parents of Andrew (an 800-gram infant born fifteen-and-a-half weeks before term, who was "in a state of painful deterioration from the start"), there is no doubt about a conflict between the parents and hospital staff. "As parents of a five-year-old daughter we know the love a mother and father feel for children," they wrote, and they wanted Andrew "to be allowed to die a natural death."[31] These wishes were opposed by the NICU staff, who were prepared to go to court for enforcement of the right to "salvage" the baby. The hospital personnel condemned the parents as "bad parents . . . intellectually tight . . . [and devoid of] feeling." The parents charged that their child was placed on a respirator "against our wishes without our consent." Andrew was "horribly trapped," they felt, "in an intensive care unit where the machinery is more sophisticated than the codes of law and ethics governing their use." The articulate and detailed account of the experience of Andrew and his parents over a six-month period filled with endless and eventually fatal medical problems is a harrowing story. The report could be entitled "The Destructiveness of Thoughtless Benevolence," for it describes in poignant language the enormity of the problem when the value domains of "victims" and "rescuers" are completely incongruent.

THE DANGER OF THE RESCUE FANTASY

How often does this kind of mismatch occur? Unfortunately we cannot say with any precision. Of course there have always been physicians opposed to saving every infant (consider the eugenics movement) and parents who believe that every infant and fetus must be saved at all costs. But the evidence suggests that a clash of values is not rare. The clues come from the testimony of experts in different fields ("At this conference [on childbirth technology] differing disciplinary outlooks gave rise to vigorous debate; genuine differences in values underlined significant areas of disagreement"[32] and from questionnaire responses by parents.[33] Surveys of the fate of infants after leaving NICUs indicate that the graduates (many of whom are born after an unwanted pregnancy[34]) incur a relatively high risk of neglect, abuse, and death.[35] There is a strong suspicion that this dismal state of affairs is due, in no small part, to what has been termed a "continuum of caretaking casualty"—when parents with marginal financial and emotional resources are overwhelmed by the survival of a sickly or malformed neonate, the situation becomes a prescription for disaster.[36] Ann Oakley's recent studies of the attitudes of women during transition to the role of motherhood suggest that childbirth—even when there are no medical complications—is often viewed as a mixed blessing: a sample of first-time, largely middle-class, London mothers frequently found the experience disappointing, and the *majority* felt angry and violent toward the new baby at some time in the postpartum period.[37]

We tend to regard anything less than whole-hearted commitment of parents to every new child as a clear sign of a psychologic disorder. But we forget that the social goal of rescuing all human offspring is a relatively recent idea.[38] And this notion, which represents a kind of extremism that might be called Reverse Social Darwinism, has not been ratified by any formal action. On the contrary, as E.M. Bates has pointed out, no extensive and continuing communication has taken place between physicians and the rest of society on this issue.[39] Society has not sanctioned the assumption of authority by those who do not live day-to-day with the long-term consequences of decisions made in neonatal matters.

Doctor Christian's statement concerning medicine's moral mission—"It is not sufficient that the medical profession should set up a standard of morality for themselves, but the people are to be educated up to it"—led me at the beginning of the intensive care movement (and leads its practitioners today) to the conviction that the medical community is doing the "right" thing. But I have become alarmed about a medical attitude that seems to regard anything less than an all-out effort to prolong the earthly existence of every human life, no matter how fragile, as a return to the practice of unrestrained infanticide. "Rescuers" justify their heroic actions with narrowly interpreted legal and theologic arguments even when their wholehearted dedication is not matched by an equal commitment on the part of parents and the community. The rescue fantasy of many physicians is not necessarily shared by most people in contemporary society. Many view unrestrained perinatal actions as short-sighted: NICU heroics may conflict with parents' interpretations of what constitutes proper social responsibility. (Andrew's parents' assessment included an estimate of his probable future, which they weighed against the happiness of their entire family.)

When ideal solutions are sought on issues for which there is no humane resolution, outcomes are often widely destructive.[40] E. Hey recently remarked, "Parents often tell me that they dread severe handicap in a young child more than death itself. In addition they often fear that medical and nursing staff will not recognize and respect these feelings."[41]

Is the new therapeutic mode of social control, in fact, a moral enterprise? Does it, on balance, further the interest of all those affected? "Medicine has nudged aside the more traditional institutions [religion and law] concerned with social control," I.K. Zola has written. "[It] is becoming the new repository of truth, the place where absolute and often final judgments are made by supposedly morally neutral and objective experts."[42] The troublesome issues concerning treatment decisions for enfeebled neonates will not go away; indeed, they are growing in importance with medicine's increasing technologic competence and the proliferation of NICUs. The conflicts deserve wide discussion, particularly with respect to achieving a proper balance of power between parents and physicians in decision-making.

I believe it was Alexis de Toqueville who warned that human institutions are, by nature, so imperfect that to destroy them it is only necessary to carry out the underlying ideas to their logical extreme. In its determination to rescue every neonate, regardless of the prognosis or the parents' feelings, the medical profession may be losing its credibility.

REFERENCES

1. Erbe RW: Genetic Disorders. *In* Wechsler H, et al: Horizons of Health. Cambridge, Harvard University Press, 1977.
2. Henshaw S, Forrest JD, Sullivan AU, Tietze C: Abortion in the United States, 1978–1979. Fam Plan Perspec 13:6–18, 1981.
3. Annotations: Whose Baby is It Anyway? Lancet 1:1284–1285, 1980.

4. Harris M: Cannibals and Kings. New York, Random House, 1977.
5. Carr-Saunders AM: The Population Problem. Oxford, Clarendon Press, 1922.
6. Isaiah 57:5
7. Cohen AE: A Jewish View toward Therapeutic Abortion and the Related Problems of Artificial Insemination and Contraception. *In* Rosen H (ed): Abortion in America. Boston, Beacon Press, 1967.
8. Langer WL: Infanticide: A Historical Survey. Hist Child Q 1:353–365, 1974.
9. Sandars TC (transl.): The Institutes of Justinian. Chicago, Callaghan & Co., 1876.
10. Singer P: Practical Ethics. Cambridge, Cambridge University Press, 1979.
11. Langer WL: Infanticide.
12. Sandars TC: The Institutes of Justinian.
13. Lecky WEH: A History of European Morals from Augustus to Charlemagne. New York, Arno Press, 1975.
14. Langer WL: Infanticide.
15. Piers MW: Infanticide Past and Present. New York, WW Norton & Co., 1978.
16. Langer WL: Checks on Population Growth: 1750–1850. Sci Amer 226:93–99, 1972. Also Kellum BA: Infanticide in England in the Later Middle Ages. Hist Child Q 1:367–388, 1974. Also Trexler RC: Infanticide in Florence: New Sources and First Results. Hist Child Q 1:98–115, 1973.
17. Langer WL: Infanticide.
18. Radbill S: A History of Child Abuse and Infanticide. *In* Kempe CH, Helfer R: The Battered Child, 3rd ed. Chicago, University of Chicago Press, 1980.
19. Walker N: Crime and Insanity in England. Edinburgh, Edinburgh University Press, 1968.
20. Damme C: Infanticide: The Worth of an Infant under Law. Med Hist 22:1–24, 1978.
21. Dworkin R: Taking Rights Seriously. Cambridge, Harvard University Press, 1977.
22. Singer P: Practical Ethics.
23. Ryan WB: Infanticide: Its Law, Prevalence, Prevention and History. London, J. Churchill, 1862.
24. Mohr JC: Abortion in America: The Origins of National Policy. New York, Oxford University Press, 1978.
25. Dunham E: Evolution of Premature Infant Care. Ann Paediatr Fenniae 3:170–184, 1957.
26. Ballantyne JW: The Problems of the Premature Infant. Lancet 1:1196–1200, 1902.
27. Budin P: Le Nourisson. Paris, Octave Doin. English translation by Maloney WJ: The Nursling. London, Caxton Publishing Co., 1907.
28. Silverman WA: Incubator-baby Side-shows. Pediatrics 64:127–141, 1979.
29. Silverman WA: Retrolental Fibroplasia: A Modern Parable. New York, Grune & Stratton, 1980.
30. Henahan J: 80% of Preemies in Follow-up Essentially Normal by Age 2. Med Trib 20:1–20, 1979.
31. Stinson R, Stinson P: On the Death of a Baby. Atl Month 244:64–72, 1979.
32. Steinfels MO: New Childbirth Technology: A Clash of Values. Hast Cent Rep 9–12, Feb 1978.
33. Riley EMD: What Do Women Want?—The Questions of Choice in the Conduct of Labour. *In* Chard T., Richards M: Benefits and Hazards of the New Obstetrics. London, Spastics Intern Med Publ, 1977.
34. Kaplan D, Mason E: Maternal Reactions to Premature Birth Viewed as an Emotional Disorder. Am J Orthopsych 30:539–547, 1960.

35. Elmer E: Children in Jeopardy. Pittsburgh, University of Pittsburgh Press, 1967. Also Skinner A, Castle R: Seventy-eight Battered Children: A Retrospective Study. London, Thomas Knight & Co., 1969. Also Kulkarni P, Hall RT, Rhodes PG, Sheehan ME: Postneonatal Mortality in Infants Admitted to a Neonatal Intensive Care Unit. Pediatrics 62:178–183, 1978.

36. Sameroff AJ, Chandler MJ: Reproductive Risk and the Continuum of Caretaking Casualty. *In* Horowitz FD (ed): Review of Child Development Research 4:187–244, 1975.

37. Oakley A: Women Confined. Toward A Sociology of Childbirth. New York, Schocken Books, 1980.

38. DeMause L: The History of Childhood. New York, The Psychohistory Press, 1974.

39. Bates EM: The Implications of Semantics for Developments in Medical Technology and the Fatal Consequences of Semantic Ignorance. Et cetera 37:25–32, 1980.

40. Marris P: Loss and Change. New York, Pantheon, 1974.

41. Hey E: Retrolental Fibroplasia as One Index of Perinatally Acquired Handicap. *In* Chalmers I, McIlwaine G: Perinatal Audit and Surveillance. London, Royal College of Obstetrics and Gynaecology, 1980.

42. Zola IK: Medicine as an Institution of Social Control. Soc Rev 20:487–504, 1972.

Norman Fost, M.D., Ph.D.

4

ETHICAL ISSUES IN THE TREATMENT OF CRITICALLY ILL NEWBORNS

A newborn with a serious birth defect, or one whose future is clouded by acquired illness, sometimes confronts parents and physicians with a tragic choice. On the one hand, there is an instinct to preserve life and maximize the infant's potential, however limited it may be. On the other hand, it often seems that such efforts may cause great suffering and harm for the family, and sometimes for the child as well. Participants in such a drama must choose whether to prolong the infant's life, or to act in a way that will shorten its life, whether by passive or active means.

Like many other ethical dilemmas in modern medicine, this one is a product of advances in technology. When techniques did not exist to keep such infants alive, there was no decision to make. It is the possibility of maintaining desperately ill patients for longer and longer periods that forces doctors and others to choose whether or not to use such techniques. It is no longer possible to avoid "playing God," if that means interfering with nature, for virtually every newborn is the beneficiary of some meddling with nature, whether it be heating the building, placing silver nitrate drops in the eyes, feeding through a synthetic nipple, or using a mechanical respirator.

At the other extreme, it seems to me that it is not feasible to declare

Reprinted by courtesy of Pediatric Annals 10:16, 1981.

that all human life is sacred and therefore warrants being preserved forever. Most of us can imagine some life not worth living, and intensive care units are increasingly populated, for prolonged periods, with patients whose prospects for meaningful life do not seem to warrant intensive care, or even minimal care. To use one extreme example, almost no one would advocate medical treatment of a child with severe anencephaly and absent kidneys.

The challenge, therefore, is to abandon slogans and find an ethically acceptable middle ground. It is the business of ethics to find justifications for actions. The alternative is to believe that actions do not require justifications, but this would be an anarchic state in which all actions would be permissible. The purpose of this chapter is to examine the various justifications that have been proposed for allowing some critically ill newborns to die, and to test their rationality and consistency.

Two presumptions are stated:

1. There is a widely shared presumption in the United States in favor of preserving human life. This is reflected in our constitution, laws, customs, and the various religious beliefs of our citizens. The great majority of people believe life is preferable to death, even when that life is accompanied by impairment or suffering. There is also an expectation that the medical profession will generally reflect this value and act to preserve life. While one could take a neutral position on whether life or death is preferred, I will start with the assumption that life should be preserved. The burden for justification, therefore, should fall on the person who advocates a course of action intended to result in death.
2. I do not believe it is acceptable to propose that everyone should live in this world forever. Since everyone can imagine some life that is not worth living, and presumably believes it is ethically justified to let such a patient die, it should be possible to state this justification in a generalizable way.

I review three common justifications for allowing a seriously ill newborn to die and suggest that they are seriously flawed. Finally, I propose a fourth justification that might better withstand scrutiny. Before getting into these substantive ethical issues, I would make one final prefatory observation about the hazards of words and labels in this area.

THE HAZARDS OF LABELS "HOPELESSLY ILL," "TERMINALLY ILL," "NONVIABLE"

The patients about whom these discussions arise sometimes are labeled "hopelessly" or "terminally" ill or "nonviable." The meaning of these phrases is often vague, and they can have powerful effects on decisions, becoming self-fulfilling prophecies.[1] Physicians may be biased toward poor prognostic statements, which further interferes with rational assessment.[2] Two examples illustrate the point.

In 1964, when I was an intern and confronted with the dilemma of whether to resuscitate a 900-gm newborn, a senior neonatologist suggested there was no duty to do so since the baby was "nonviable." It was apparently meant as an empiric observation that no baby that size had ever survived for an extended period at that hospital. Since other hospitals were apparently successfully resuscitating some infants of that size at that time, they presumably did not take the empiric statement of "nonviability" to be ethically persuasive and attempted to push back the frontier of viability. Whether or not such an infant lived depended, in some large measure, on attitudes and decisions of those around the patient. There was nothing intrinsically nonviable about such an infant. The label, however, could put the patient in a category where treatment would be withheld and the label would therefore determine a course of action which was fatal.

An even more hopeless condition than prematurity was a clinical state known in the late 1950s as "death." The physiologic correlate was cardiorespiratory arrest, now simply known as "the most serious arrhythmia imaginable."[3] Patients with cardiac arrest are not only no longer hopeless, they are, like 1000-gm infants, successfully treated in many cases. The cure—external cardiac massage—had been described in the nineteenth century, but lay fallow until rediscovered in the mid twentieth century.[4] We now define death in other ways, again illustrating that even something that sounds as hopeless as death may be neither hopeless nor terminal, but dependent on the knowledge and attitudes of the medical staff.

The relevance for critically ill newborns is the importance of avoiding inappropriate labels which lead to ethically unjustifiable actions.[5] Two examples of infants with "Do Not Resuscitate" orders based on premature designations of "hopeless" will suffice:

- an infant with severe neonatal seizures, lethargy, and a markedly abnormal electroencephalogram. Reduction of phenobarbital was followed by clinical improvement. The seizures abated and, on two-year follow-up, she was normal.
- an infant with diagnoses of "intractable" bronchopulmonary dysplasia, infantile-type polycystic kidneys, and "inoperable" congenital heart disease. The latter was eventually shown to be a patent ductus, the lung disease was resolved, and the polycystic kidneys were shown to be adult-type.[6]

Good ethics start with good facts, and sound ethical reasoning will not rescue a decision predicated on false assumptions.[7] Clinical decisions will always be based on imperfect data, but in the presence of great uncertainty—which can be reduced by consultation, a therapeutic trial, or a limited period of observation—the best course usually is to avoid making an irreversible decision based on wrong information.

We now turn to the various proposals that have been used as justifications for withholding care from seriously ill newborns.

DISTINCTIONS BETWEEN ORDINARY AND EXTRAORDINARY MEANS

It is commonly said that we ought to provide ordinary care for all patients, but that we have no obligation to use extraordinary means to keep a patient alive. Appealing though this guideline may be, it founders in practice because of the difficulty in defining the words in a useful or consistent way.

One noncontroversial definition of extraordinary would be "heroic" or "beyond the call of duty." Clarity, in this case, is achieved by circularity, for we must define our duty before we can know what is beyond its call. If by duty we mean all those things that are ordinary, or those things that are not extraordinary, all we have established is a circular statement that there is no duty to do things which are beyond the call of duty. This is amusing but not helpful.

Another proposed definition of extraordinary is "expensive." This tells us what is meant, but not in a way that is useful, since expensive is another vague and relative term. For some, one day in the hospital is expensive; for others, it is a trivial cost. Some define expensive as "more than a person can afford," but this would entitle the rich to more medical care than the poor. Moreover, even if we could agree on a definition of expensive that was not discriminatory, it is not clear why it would justify nontreatment or why we would want a system in which such a principle were consistently applied. Everyone might agree, for example, that an appendectomy is expensive, but that alone would not justify withholding such an operation from a patient.

Some define extraordinary as "unnatural," but this includes too much. Virtually every newborn is dependent on unnatural support for survival, whether it be heat, artificial light, prepared formula, or more complex technology. Confining our obligations to natural means would limit newborn care to whole milk and bonfires.

Finally, some would define "extraordinary" as "that which is unlikely to benefit the patient." Under this definition, even simple treatment, such as food, water, or heat, could be considered extraordinary if the patient's condition were irreversible. This objection can be overcome by combining some concept of excessive expense or discomfort with the notion of "no likely benefit." The more serious problem is in defining benefit. Some would use this definition to justify withholding medical care that would otherwise be considered ordinary from a child with Down's syndrome, on the argument that the retardation will not be alleviated or the child benefited by such treatment. Using the definition this way, any treatment for a medical complication in a retarded person would be considered extraordinary. If the intended benefit is restricted to the medical condition which prompted the treatment (eg, intestinal obstruction in the case of the child with Down's syndrome and duodenal atresia, or ventriculitis in the case of hydrocephalus), there is still ambiguity as to what would constitute a benefit. There would be disagreement, for example, about whether extending the life of a retarded person by several weeks or months constitutes a benefit. Judgment on such matters is likely to be arbitrary and not resolvable by defining "extraordinary" in any consistent way.

Some would say they cannot define the terms, but that they can use them operationally in a consistent way. A respirator, for example, frequently comes to mind as an example *par excellence* of extraordinary means. A novice might ask, in response, whether that would permit withholding a respirator from an otherwise normal postoperative patient who needed five minutes of ventilatory support. Most would say that such a treatment would be ordinary and therefore required. This suggests that there is nothing intrinsic to the technology that is extraordinary, but rather that it would be extraordinary to use such means in certain cases. It appears to be something about the patient that makes use of technologies extraordinary, even though they are considered ordinary in other settings.

Extraordinary means, therefore, appears to be a term used when a physician believes it is appropriate to withhold medical care from a patient, even though the means are called *ordinary* in other settings. The crucial variable is something about the patient, not something about the means, and the phrase should probably be changed to "extraordinary patient." This interpretation is supported by a survey of pediatricians in which many considered repair of duodenal atresia in an otherwise normal child "ordinary means," but called the same operation on a child with Down's syndrome "extraordinary means."[8] The means are the same in both cases, and cannot be ordinary in one and not the other. What is presumably meant by the respondents is that there is something about patients with Down's syndrome that would make it extraordinary to do an operation which, in other patients, would be ordinary.

ALLOCATION OF SCARCE RESOURCES

A second justification offered for withholding treatment from newborns is based on the claim that to use limited resources on a defective child is a misallocation of scarce supplies, personnel, and equipment. It is unarguable that all resources are limited, and that to provide services for one patient often means that some other person will do without. It is therefore unavoidable that at some level, decisions have to be made about how to distribute benefits and burdens. I do not intend here to discuss in detail the merits of various proposals for allocation at the *macro* level. I am primarily addressing proposals to let a specific identifiable patient die (in the absence of a clear public policy) based on a personal opinion that the patient represented a misallocation of scarce resources.

There are three reasons why withholding treatment on these grounds may be criticized.

1. To say that spending resources in this way is a bad allocation is to imply that to spend them in some other way is good or morally preferable. While there are reasons to prefer some allocation schemes to others, there is often no morally compelling argument provided in favor of one scheme. It is difficult to find a persuasive moral argument for spending limited funds on defense rather than medical care, or medical care rather than job training or education. Even within health, there is no morally compelling reason for preferring prevention to crisis intervention or research. Even if there were limited funds for crisis intervention, it is not clear why the physician should feel a higher duty to some future patient with whom he has no relationship, than to a patient presently under his care and whom he has already agreed to treat.

2. Even if there were a morally compelling argument for withholding treatment from defective newborns in favor of future normal children, it is unpredictable whether that reallocation would in fact occur. Past experience with such reallocation arguments, such as during the Vietnam war, suggests that liberated funds enter the same marketplace as all revenues and are as likely to end up in highway construction as in health. If the reason for withholding treatment from Patient X is to conserve funds so that hypothetical Patient Y might be better treated, there should be a reasonable expectation that the funds will in fact be used for Patient Y. That assurance is rarely available.

3. Even if it were conceded that it would be appropriate and fair for society to use its resources in a way that discriminated against the least-advantaged members, it would not follow that it is appropriate for a physician to make that decision at the bedside. Physicians are neither competent nor authorized to allocate community resources. They are expected to provide the best medical service available, within the constraints set by society, but it would appear to be beyond the physician's job to decide which members of the community deserve treatment and which do not. An analogy can be made with the case of a fire-truck driver choosing which houses he will save by putting out the fire, basing his decision on his personal view that saving the occupants of one house represents a better allocation of community resources.

Different arguments would arise in the case of triage, which refers to a situation in which only one of two patients can be treated and the physician *must* choose which one to treat. This is not a common situation in pediatric practice today. The more typical situation is that it is possible to treat the patient, but an argument is made that one ought not to provide that treatment. This is different from the setting in which someone must die because it is impossible to treat all.

PARENTAL DESIRES

Probably the most common reason given for withholding life-saving treatment from a seriously ill newborn is based on deference to parental wishes.[9-12] To give one person life-and-death power over another suggests a special relationship, since we generally do not believe that "one person's life can be subject to another person's desires."[13] Three models of the parent-child relationship have been proposed: ownership, trusteeship, and equal rights.

Ownership.

One might postulate that the parent-child relationship was one of ownership. This was a prevailing view in Western civilization for most of its history. Infanticide was widely tolerated in England and France until late in the nineteenth century.[14,15] This view is no longer prevalent. Child-abuse and -neglect laws are one reflection of the widely held view that the state should intervene when parents act in a way that threatens a child's life or safety.[16]

Trusteeship.

This model acknowledges that the parents have broad authority over the child's life in such matters as training in religion, education, and behavior, but also upholds the State's responsibility to intervene when parental decisions present a clear and present danger to the child's life.

Equal Rights.

The third conceivable model would be based on the belief that parents and children have equal rights, with no presumption of either class having priority when their interests conflict. This would leave unresolved the exceptionally rare case in which the child's continued existence presented a threat to the life of the parent, but would suggest that the child's right to life would take precedence over a parental interest in avoiding lesser problems such as discomfort, economic burden, or stigma. If two persons are of equal status, it would not be permissible to let one die simply because his existence would be likely to cause discomfort or to burden the other.

Postulating that the child's rights are equal to the parents' would not, however, lead to the conclusion that all children should be kept alive. There comes a point in virtually every person's life when he no longer has an interest in living, when his best interests are served by letting him die. For some, that point may come very early. We now turn to this justification for letting a newborn die.

EUTHANASIA IN THE CHILD'S INTEREST

I have urged that arguments for discontinuing care based on ordinary-extraordinary distinctions, societal-economic benefits, and parental wishes do not by themselves suffice to justify such action. If, however, a patient of any age has no interest in living, or if that patient's interests seem to be best served by letting him die, then it is not only permissible to let such a patient die, but it might also be obligatory. The remaining difficulty is to define those circumstances in which a child's interest would be best served by death, or to define an acceptable process for making such a judgment.

McCormick has suggested a substantive criterion for discontinuing care of a severely damaged newborn: the potential for human relationships.[18] Jonsen also relied heavily on this factor, among others, as being crucial.[19] Such a standard would justify withholding care from an anencephalic, and presumably other vegetatively retarded infants. It would presumably not justify discontinuation of care of infants with such conditions as Down's syndrome, meningomyelocoele, and intraventricular hemorrhage. It is this group—destined to be retarded and/or severely handicapped—that constitutes the more common problem for the practicing pediatrician, the majority of whom would defer to a parental request for discontinuation of care.[8,20] Such infants do not fit McCormick's or Jonsen's criteria for passive euthanasia, and justification must therefore be sought on other grounds.

Goldstein and his associates have suggested that parents should have the authority to withhold lifesaving treatment from their children if it is unlikely the child will ". . . have either a life worth living or a life of relatively normal growth. . . ."[21] When reasonable people disagree about whether the life is worth living, he advocates leaving the judgment to the parents. This is not quite the same as allowing a child to die simply because of parental whim or discretion. Rather, it states a standard which must be met before care can be withheld—"a life not worth living"—and suggests that parents are best situated to make that judgment, or in the absence of consensus, as competent as anyone else to decide. In theory, this would justify depriving someone of his right to life if two conditions were met: the parents wanted the person to die, and reasonable people disagreed about whether his/her life was worth living. In practice, it resulted in the denial of medically recommended lifesaving heart surgery to a 10-year-old boy who, by all accounts, was enjoying life as much as any normal person his age.[22] Given the certainty of a slow, painful death without surgery and a 90% chance of normal cardiac function with surgery, it seems unlikely that a competent person with many decades of life ahead would choose for premature death. By Goldstein's analysis, however, because reasonable people disagree about whether a retarded person's life is worth living, the parents were given authority to deny the child standard therapy for his medical condition.

In the absence of agreement on substantive criteria, some have sought a procedural approach for maximizing the probability that the infant's best interest will be served. A theoretical basis for such an approach comes from "ideal observer theory," which states that an action can be considered right if it would be approved by an ideal observer with the following qualities: (1) omniscience, meaning access to all the relevant available facts; (2) omnipercipience, meaning an ability to imagine vividly the feelings of others involved; (3) disinterest, meaning having no vested interest in the outcome;

(4) dispassion, meaning not being overwhelmed by feelings so strong as to cloud critical thinking; and (5) consistency, meaning similar cases would be decided similarly.[23]

Commitment to this process would seem to disqualify individuals as proxies for the child. Parents often fall short by lacking relevant prognostic information and by sometimes being overwhelmed with negative feelings toward the child. And most important, they may have overt conflicts of interest, particularly when they see the child's continued interest as being a threat to their own wellbeing.[24] Similarly, physicians may often be less than "ideal observers." A commitment to pushing back the frontier of viability, a tendency to accept death as failure, or even an overt research interest are examples of conflicts of interest and emotional biases which may cloud critical thinking.

Since no one person possesses these Godlike qualities, it has been suggested that a process might better emulate the ideal observer than would an individual.[7,25] A decision resulting from a process that embodied these concepts would not necessarily be right, but it would be more likely to be approved by an ideal observer. It is these considerations that have led to the recent interest in hospital-based ethics committees and the increasing involvement of courts in decisions about life and death.[26–30]

This intrusion into the doctor-patient relationship is accompanied by its own unwelcome costs, including loss of control by physicians and families. Thus far, the law usually has not intruded itself without a request from a physician, but there are potential legal hazards for physicians and others, including a charge of negligent homicide.[31] In 1975, Dr. Edelin was found guilty of negligent manslaughter for failing to resuscitate a possibly viable fetus following a legal midtrimester hysterotomy abortion. His conviction was overturned on technical grounds, but the court did state that it would have been upheld if it had been clear that the infant had been born alive.[32] More recently, a prosecution has been initiated against parents and a physician who allegedly attempted to starve a pair of Siamese twins sharing a common intestinal tract.[33]

All other cases (Quinlan, Saikewicz, Fox, Springs, Becker) have been triggered by a request for judicial guidance from physicians or others involved with the care of the patient. No case involving a defective newborn has reached an appellate court, and related cases relay a mixed message. Some, involving decisions by parents to withhold standard treatment for acute lymphocytic leukemia, have found such decisions unacceptable and ordered treatment over the parents' objections.[34] In contrast, a California appellate court upheld a decision by parents to withhold lifesaving heart surgery from a 10-year-old boy with Down's syndrome, despite their estrangement from the child since the newborn period and his failure to recognize them as his psychologic parents.[19] Like it or not, we are probably at the beginning of an era of increasing legal involvement in such decisions. It is unclear what limits, if any, will be put on the traditional discretion granted to physicians and parents.

CONCLUSION

A decision to withhold lifesaving medical care from a human being is an ethical issue of profound importance. To deprive a person of the fundamental right to life requires justification beyond personal preference. It is suggested that the only compelling reason for letting a child die is when there are reasonable grounds for concluding that it is in the child's best interests to die. Since parents and physicians, acting alone, may not be well situated to ascertain and represent the child's interests, a commitment to a process that more closely approximates an "ideal observer" may be preferred.

REFERENCES

1. Fost N, Chudwin D, Wikler D: The limited moral significance of fetal viability. Hastings Cent. Rep. 10:10–13, 1980.
2. Siegler M: Pascal's wager and the hanging of crepe. N Engl J Med 293: 853–857, 1975.
3. Nadas A: Pediatric Cardiology, 2nd ed. Philadelphia, W B Saunders Co., 1964.
4. Kouewenhoven WB, Jude JR, Knickerbocker CG: Closed-chest cardiac massage. JAMA 173:1064–1067, 1960.
5. Pasternak JF, Volpe JJ: Full recovery from prolonged brainstem failure following intraventricular hemorrhage. J Pediatr 95:1046–1049, 1979.
6. Fost N: Proxy consent for seriously ill newborns. *In* Smith D (ed) No Rush to Judgment: Essays on Medical Ethics, Bloomington, Ind., The Poynter Foundation, 1978.
7. Fost N: Good ethics start with good facts. *In* Davidson F (ed)Making Clinical Judgments, Carbondale, Ill., Southern Illinois University Press, (in press).
8. Shaw A, Randolph JG, Manard B: Ethical issues in pediatric surgery: A nationwide survey of pediatricians and pediatric surgeons. Pediatrics 60: 588–599, 1977.
9. Duff RS, Campbell AGM: Moral and ethical dilemmas in the special-care nursery. N Engl J Med 289:890–894, 1973.
10. Kelsey B: Which infants shall live? An interview with Raymond Duff. Hastings Cent Rep 5:5–8, 1975.
11. Duff RS: On deciding the care of severely handicapped or dying persons, with particular reference to infants. Pediatrics 57:487–492, 1976.
12. Duff R: Counseling families and deciding care of severely defective children. Pediatrics 67:315–320, 1981.
13. Gustafson J: Mongolism, parental desires, and the right to life. Persp Biol Med 16:529–557, 1973.
14. DeMause L: The History of Childhood. New York, Psychohistory Press, 1974.
15. Langer WI: Infanticide: A historical survey. Hist Child Q. 1:353–388, 1974.
16. Paulsen MG: The law and abused children. *In* Helfer RF, Kempe CH (eds): The Battered Child. 2nd ed. Chicago, University of Chicago Press, 1974.
17. Wald M: State intervention on behalf of neglected children: A search for realistic standards. Stanford Law Rev 27:985, 1975.
18. McCormick RA: To save or let die: The dilemma of modern medicine. JAMA 229:172–176, 1974.

19. Jonsen AR, et al: Critical issues in newborn intensive care: A conference report and policy proposal. Pediatrics 55:756–768, 1975.
20. Todres ID, et al: Pediatricians' attitudes affecting decision-making in defective newborns. Pediatrics 60:197–201, 1977.
21. Goldstein J, Freud A, Solnit AJ: Before the Best Interest of the Child. New York, The Free Press, 1979.
22. Annas GJ: Denying the rights of the retarded: The Phillip Becker case. Hastings Cent Rep 9:18–20, 1979.
23. Firth R: Ethical absolutism and the ideal observer. J Philos Phenomen Res 12:317, 1952.
24. Fost N: Counselling families who have a child with severe congenital anomaly. Pediatrics 67:321–324, 1981.
25. Fost N: Ethical problems in pediatrics. Curr Probl Pediatr 6:1–31, 1976.
26. Optimum care for hopelessly ill patients. A report of the critical care committee of the Massachusetts General Hospital. N Engl J Med 295:362–364, 1976.
27. Baron CH: Assuring detached but passionate investigation and decision: The role of guardians ad litem in *Saikewicz*-type cases. Am J Law Med 4:111–130, 1978.
28. Annas G: Quinlan, Saikewicz and now Brother Fox. Hastings Cent Rep 10: 20–21, 1980.
29. Annas G: Quality of life in the courts. Earle Spring in fantasyland. Hastings Cent Rep 10:9–10, 1980.
30. Robertson JA: Legal norms and procedures for withholding care from incompetent patients: The role of law in passive euthanasia. *In* Abernethy V (ed): Frontiers in Medical Ethics: Applications in a Medical Setting. Cambridge, Mass., Ballinger, 1980.
31. Robertson JA, Fost N: Passive euthanasia of defective newborns: Legal considerations. J Pediatr 88:883–889, 1976.
32. Robertson JA: After Edelin: Little guidance. Hastings Cent Rep 7:15–17, 1977.
33. Wadler J: Siamese twins parents charged. Washington Post. June 11, 1981.
34. Horwitz FT: Of love and laetrile: Medical decision making in a child's best interests. Am J Law Med 5:271–294, 1979.

John E. Schowalter, M.D.
Julian B. Ferholt, M.D.
Nancy M. Mann, M.S.W.

5

THE ADOLESCENT PATIENT'S DECISION TO DIE

Those who are treating a severely ill patient who decides to die are faced with an agonizing dilemma. The problem is magnified when life can be sustained for a significant period if the patient accepts dependence on a drug, a procedure, or a machine. A patient may, however, refuse further transfusions, another course of a cytotoxic drug, further cancer surgery or radiation, an organ transplant, renal dialysis, or an artificial organ or pacemaker. New techniques to prolong life make this problem increasingly common in situations where death is not imminent, but the quality of life is greatly impaired. In pediatrics, the problem of a patient's decision to die is complicated even more by special developmental, ethical, legal, and family considerations. There has been little discussion in the medical literature of these issues, but recently there has been editorial recognition of the need for further debate on the issues of euthanasia and the child's right to die.[1-3] The basic question to be faced is should a physician always oppose a patient's request to end his life, and if not, under what conditions should he respect or even support a patient in his decision to die? These are situations of conflict between our commitment to relieve suffering and our commitment to prolong life. Sometimes it is evident to everyone that death is imminent, the suffering severe, and that efforts to prolong life will only

Reprinted with permission of Pediatrics 51(1):97–103, Jan 1973.

prolong suffering, while at other times it is clear that the wish to die is irrationally out of proportion to the suffering. There is also, however, a very difficult middle ground. Especially in these cases patients may disagree with their parents, patient and family may disagree with the medical staff, and various members of the medical staff may disagree with each other.

On the Adolescent Ward of Yale-New Haven Hospital, the authors recently helped to treat an adolescent who chose to die. This paper is an outcome of our considerations prior to and following her death.

CASE REPORT

Karen was a 16-year-old Catholic girl, the second oldest of seven siblings. She was first hospitalized in September 1968, after a three-week course of nephrotic syndrome. She did not respond to medical management. A renal biopsy in April 1969 revealed "chronic, active glomerulonephritis," and by spring of 1970 a rapid decrease in renal function prompted the decision to plan for dialysis and transplantation. A bilateral nephrectomy was performed in August 1970, and Karen received a transplant of her father's kidney the following month. The transplant functioned quite well initially, but several months later proteinuria became increasingly severe, and suddenly in March 1971 the kidney completely ceased to function. Prior to surgery and following the transplant's failure, thrice-weekly hemodialysis was performed. Karen tolerated dialysis poorly, routinely having chills, nausea, vomiting, severe headaches, and weakness.

In April 1970 and prior to transplantation, a child psychiatrist (J.F.) was asked to evaluate the family. Karen was found to have a reactive depression, but this was considered appropriate. The father responded to his daughter's illness by immersing himself in his profession. The mother evidenced a suspiciousness of Karen's medical management that contained circumferential speech, loosening of thought associations, and an inappropriate lability of affect. Referral of the mother for psychiatric outpatient treatment was recommended by never accomplished.

The child psychiatrist was again consulted in July 1970. Karen and her parents met regularly with the social worker (N.M.) and the child psychiatrist (J.F.) prior to and after the transplant. The family did well psychologically during the immediate posttransplant period, but as Karen's new kidney failed, she became moderately depressed and the parents became increasingly distraught. Marital difficulties developed as the family could not deal directly with their disappointment at the transplant failing. The marital problems lessened with open discussion of the parents' feelings about the possible failure of the transplant.

In early April 1971, after it was clear that the kidney would never function, Karen and her parents expressed the wish to stop medical treatment and let "nature take its course." The medical staff was upset and they could not agree on the proper course of action. The social worker and psychiatrist attempted to have the girl and her family explore their decision in the hope that with further understanding of the decision, they would reject it. Most other staff members conveyed to the family that such wishes were unheard of and unacceptable and that a decision to stop treatment could never be an alternative. The family did decide to continue dialysis, medication, and diet therapy. Karen's renal incapacity returned to pretransplant levels and she returned to a socially isolated life, diet restrictions, chronic discomfort and fatigue.

On May 10, Karen was hospitalized following ten days of high fever. Three days later the transplant was removed. Its pathology resembled that of the original kidneys, and the possibility of a similar reaction forming in subsequent transplants was established.

On May 21, the arteriovenous shunt placed in Karen's arm for hemodialysis was found to be infected, and part of the vein wall was excised and the shunt revised. During this portion of the hospitalization, Karen and the parents grudgingly went along with the medical recommendations, but they continued to ponder the possibility of stopping treatment. The child psychiatrist was out of town from the end of April, and the social worker was now counseling Karen as well as her parents. On May 24, the shunt clotted closed. Karen, with her parents' agreement, refused shunt revision and any further dialysis.

Those connected with Karen's treatment were stunned by frustration and anger. They felt that the decision was immoral and unsound medically. The idea of a 16-year-old patient deciding her own fate was anathema. Karen had occasionally spoken to her parish priest. Following her decision she stopped seeing him but continued to talk with the hospital chaplain. She came to the personal conclusion that there was no such place as hell and even if there was not a heaven, nothingness would be far better than the suffering that would continue if she lived. On May 26, the child psychiatry consultant for the ward (J.S.), who was familiar with the situation from the time of the transplant, was asked to evaluate the girl. He found no evidence of psychotic thinking and was convinced that Karen had carefully thought out her decision and had grasped its implications.

The child psychiatrist and the attending ward physician (who happened to be a nephrologist) decided independently that Karen's decision was made as rationally as any such decision could be. They believed the staff had little choice but to comply with her request, making her dying as comfortable as possible and providing the opportunity through daily counseling for her to change her mind at any time. At first no other staff member agreed with the decision. Nurses, house officers, and consultants spent sleepless nights; faces were haggard, tempers short, and the ward morale, which usually ran high, was undermined. Almost daily staff meetings were held to discuss the policy toward Karen. Alternative suggestions ranged from having the courts take custody of the child and force treatment to demanding the parents to take the girl home to die so as not to taint the hospital or staff with the voluntary death. Some staff members felt they were being forced to act as accomplices to what they believed was a suicide. Much anger was expressed at the parents for participating in Karen's decision ("It's on their heads not ours"), and many voiced a belief that if the parents gave Karen back to "Medicine" that all would be well.

The attitude of the ward staff changed, however, as the bleak medical alternatives were discussed in the ward meetings and when Karen's appetite and spirits improved after she made her decision. By May 30, when a nurse from the dialysis unit visited Karen and upset her by insisting that she return to dialysis, a majority of the staff agreed with the family that this strident approach was undesirable, and the nurse was asked not to visit. Those that knew Karen the best found it easier to acquiesce to her decision than those, especially the house officers, who recently came onto the floor. This reaction was consistent with a previous finding that those who directly witness a dying patient's suffering are less eager than more remote physicians to prolong the life of the child in extremis.[4]

Karen died on June 2, with both parents at her bedside. The relative speed and peacefulness of her dying were unusual for a uremic death. Shortly before her death, she thanked the staff for what she said she knew had been a hard time for them and she told her parents she hoped they would be happy. We later learned that before her death she had written a will and had picked a burial spot near her home and near her favorite horseback-riding trail. In the final days she supported her parents as they faltered in their decision; she told her father, "Daddy, I will be happy there (in the ground) if there is no machine and they don't work on me any more." Six months later the family is proceeding through a quite normal grief sequence with a minimum of psychiatric (J.F.) and pastoral assistance.

It is clear in this case that issues of morality are entangled for the staff with feelings of omnipotence, impotence, control, and altruism. For the family also the motivations are complex and multidetermined. However, it is not our intent to discuss this case further but to use it to illustrate the dilemma facing those who care for an ill child who chooses to die. We present here a brief review of the literature and a summary of our approach to these difficult problems.

DEVELOPMENTAL CONSIDERATIONS

Although Freud stated that probably no one can ever fully comprehend his own death, a crucial consideration in evaluating a patient's wish to die is whether or not he can understand the concept of death.[5] The school of Piagetian psychology suggests that the grasping of the possibilities and limitations of one's self in relation to a finite future develop within the stage of formal operations, occurring during adolescence.[6] Other psychologists, as well as pediatric clinicians, concur.[7,8] So, it is generally agreed that by age 14 or 15 most adolescents can understand the meaning of death.

It is rare for children who have not yet reached adolescence to decide to die. When this does occur, it is likely that the child does not comprehend the meaning of death, and the real meaning of his wish must be investigated and responded to. When an adolescent decides to die, his understanding of death's meaning and permanence must also be assessed.

On the one hand, it must be kept in mind that the cognitive understanding of death can exist without the emotional maturity necessary to make final decisions regarding one's own life. On the other hand, older adolescents, like our patient, can appreciate their suffering and fatigue and can comprehend when it is likely that life will never offer any more than continued disability, doubt and suffering.

PSYCHOLOGIC REACTIONS OF STAFF

A patient's wish for death forces staff members to confront their personal mortality and sometimes a latent self-destructive wish. This experience can be very uncomfortable, and some people must react with denial. Studies have shown that physicians and medical students are often individuals with especially strong feelings about death and with strong wishes to avoid facing death.[9-13] Our society reinforces the tendency to deny death and condemn suicide. Suicide is punished by everything from life insurance nonpayment to the threat of criminal prosecution and from incarceration in a mental hospital to religious damnation. In addition, for a physician, the choosing of death by a patient represents defeat and a rebuff of his role as healer.[14]

So if, as Kasper suggests, the physician considers his own fears about death, puts them as intellectual questions, and tries to answer them for other people, a patient's decision to die can threaten the physician on both personal and professional grounds.[15]

McKegney and Lange reported on four adults in dialysis who chose to die.[16] These authors stress the importance of the staff's recognizing the possibility of a patient's wishing to die and aiding the patient to bring forth and discuss this wish before it becomes crystallized into a firm conviction. In these reported cases, the dialysis staff members continued to operate on the assumption that life was always preferable to death. When the patients did not share this value judgment, the staff became angry, accusing them of not living up to their part of the bargain. This staff reaction, which we also noted, is understandable, especially since dialysis staff seem especially to demand that patients do well in return for devoted care.[17]

As a result of these psychologic stresses, staff can react with anger, irritability, or depression, which may trigger an attempt to seek a rapid conclusion of events without proper exploration. A staff member may deny the obvious fact that a patient wishes to die and may even transmit to the family that such thoughts are not acceptable. On the other hand, he may avoid strong feelings by a too easy compliance with the wishes of the patient. If unnoticed, these psychologic reactions may interfere with the professional's ability to determine and serve the best interests of his patient.

PSYCHOLOGIC REACTIONS OF PATIENTS WITH CHRONIC RENAL DISEASE

Patients with chronic renal disease are the best studied group in terms of their reacting to a very uncomfortable, usually fatal disorder. Suicidal behavior has been one focus of this literature. In the study of one group of 14 patients, the fear of living the unsatisfactory life of the chronically ill and handicapped seemed almost as intolerable as the fear of imminent death; while in another study of 25 patients, the main concern was not in dying or living as much as "that it would be decided one way or the other quickly."[18,19] Other studies emphasize the patient's concern about the quality of his life. Abram et al, in a questionnaire study including 127 centers and involving 3478 renal dialysis patients, found that if suicides were considered as those patients who died suddenly by their own hand as well as those who died following voluntary withdrawal from the program or following refusal to adhere to the treatment regimen, the suicide rate was 400 times that of the general population.[20] If only outright suicides and deaths following withdrawal from treatment were included, the "suicide" rate was 100 times that in the general population. Although the accuracy of the percentages from such a questionnaire study is suspect, the fact that many patients with chronic renal disease do choose death over prolonged dying does seem substantiated.

Although most reports of reactions of patients with chronic kidney diseases have been in adults, cases of nonpsychotic children on dialysis who exhibited self-destructive behavior, including trying to remove their shunt, have been reported and discussed.[21,22] Reinhart's experience in Pittsburgh led him to the extreme position of seriously questioning the value of chronic dialysis or renal transplantation for children at all at this time.[23]

Many reports question the quality of life on chronic dialysis for some patients and their families. Perhaps this is an area where in our enthusiasm for a new procedure we frequently underestimate the psychologic suffering of patients. In our opinion, psychologic services to these patients are essential, and indications for the procedure must include psychosocial factors. No matter how useful it is to have the statistics of other patients' experiences with a particular disease, every evaluation must consider the patient's specific handicaps in relation to the personal values of each family, the developmental stage of each patient, and the services in the community available to support and improve the quality of the patient's life.

MORAL AND LEGAL CONSIDERATIONS

A complete discussion of the ethical implications of this type of case could be the subject of a long philosophic treatise; we can only outline a few major considerations. Moral analysis deals with the justification for behavior; it attempts to analyze how right, virtuous, or excellent the action is. The judgment may be made in relation to the ideals of a particular person, the mores of a particular time and place, or the imperatives of an ethical philosophy. The approach taken will determine the choices which seem possible, and the values which are emphasized or ignored in an analysis can determine the judgment. Furthermore, the complexity increases in our modern society, where values differ greatly and change rapidly. In any case, we must contend with the values of the patient, the family, the medical staff, and society as a whole.

Honoring a child's wish to die can be viewed as committing a homicide, abetting a suicide, or administering euthanasia, depending on the circumstances and one's philosophy. Euthanasia is commonly understood to mean only actively causing a patient's death rather than passively allowing it to occur, and suicide is commonly understood to mean taking one's own life rather than allowing death to occur by "natural" causes. Fletcher, however, categorizes euthanasia as voluntary (depending on the patient's knowledge and wishes) and as active or passive (depending on whether death is hastened by action or inaction).[24,25] Karen's death would be considered passive, voluntary euthanasia. That is, the physicians chose to honor an informed rational choice to die by inaction based on the judgment that the child accurately perceived her own best interests.

Most physicians' ethics oppose actively causing death. In Williams' questionnaire study of 33 members of the Association of Professors of Medicine and the Association of American Physicians, 87% voted in favor of passive euthanasia and 80% have practiced it, while 85% of the physicians opposed active euthanasia.[26] In a study of 418 physicians in Seattle, 59% favored passive euthanasia (after having obtained a signed request from relatives), and 31% favored active euthanasia.[27] Morison and Kass have recently debated whether or not it is correct to distinguish ethically between intent and means.[28,29] Intent in all euthanasia is the same, but the means differ.

Although rarely prosecuted, euthanasia is a crime in America. Passive euthanasia makes a physician vulnerable to prosecution for clinical neglect; active euthanasia makes a physician vulnerable to prosecution for homicide. Recent attempts to legalize euthanasia have failed in Great Britain.

Passive, voluntary and even active, nonvoluntary euthanasia are occasionally performed for the terminally ill child or the monstrously deformed newborn. Voluntary euthanasia for a child who is chronically but not terminally ill is rare but may become increasingly common with the increasing number of patients' lives being sustained by artificial and often uncomfortable and expensive means. Karen, for example, was not terminal at the time of the decision, because dialysis could have prolonged her life for a considerable period of time.

Those against legalized euthanasia emphasize its possible misuses and associate it with totalitarian eugenics. They stress that approval of euthanasia would contradict the physician's commitment to heal and undermine the confidence of all patients in their physicians. The possibility of a mistaken diagnosis or of a cure being discovered during the patient's prolonged dying are also cited as objections to the practice of euthanasia. Religious opposition to all forms of euthanasia rests on belief in the divine nature of suffering or the exclusive right of God to determine the time of death.

Nonmedical writers tend to favor a policy that would allow the dying a quick, painless end. Fielding commented that "it hath been often said that it is not death, but dying, which is terrible."[30] Sophocles put it, "For death is not the worst but when one wants to die and cannot even have that death."[31] Supposedly, after a colleague proposed amputation of his toes, the great French surgeon Ambroise Paré replied, "I prefer to die by the hand of God." An example closer to home both historically and geographically was the planned death of Percy Williams Bridgman, the distinguished philosopher of science at Harvard, who when dying of cancer wrote: "I would like to take advantage of the situation in which I find myself to establish a general principle, namely, that when the ultimate end is inevitable as it now appears to be, the individual has a right to ask his doctor to end it for him."[32] When this request was not granted and he had ended his own life, a note was found which read: "It isn't decent for Society to make a man do this thing himself."

Those who accept limited euthanasia try to define guidelines. Catholic moral theology makes the useful distinction between ordinary and extraordinary means of actions. Pope Pius XII stated that "it is not obligatory for physicians to use extraordinary means to prolong life indefinitely in hopeless cases."[33] Gerald Kelly, the Catholic Theologian, wrote that "extraordinary means of preserving life are all medicines, treatments and operations which cannot be obtained or used without excessive expense, pain, or other inconvenience for the patient or for others or which, if used, would not offer reasonable hope of benefit to the patient."[34] Gustafson points out one difficulty with the definition of "extraordinary"; the same procedure may be ordinary for one patient but extraordinary for another, depending on the extent of the problems the patient has.[35]

A second difficulty in using the ordinary-extraordinary distinction as a guideline is the interpretation of the word hopeless. An assessment of hopelessness includes the patient's nearness to death and the amount of his suffering, as well as the physician's attitudes toward physical suffering, psychologic suffering, and the relative importance of quality to quantity of life. Gustafson warns that in assessing the quality of life, no single quality can be allowed to be considered determinative. We need to encompass the variety, complexity, and interplay of the qualities we value. Major considerations might include self-determination, happiness, satisfaction in fulfilling even limited goals, and providing occasion for meaningful experiences for others, both distressing and joyful.[35]

Aside from the fact that death was not imminent for Karen, another unique feature is Karen's age. The families' obligations are undefined in childhood euthanasia. Literature on human experimentation, although a very difficult situation, suggests that the rights of parents should be limited if risk or harm to the child is possible.[36,37] The child's consent is usually considered increasingly necessary with increasing age, but some argue that even if parent and child consent, only therapeutic research should be permissible.[38,39] Others believe informed consent can be considered complete only when accompanied by some sort of ethical counseling. Even more difficult than when parents and child agree on a wish to end treatment are situations when the parents, but not the child, want to stop life-sustaining support or when the child wishes death, while the parents disagree. Although the study of such dilemmas is too complex to tackle here, the courts could probably be used to safeguard the first type of patient, while a child adamantly bent on self-destruction can probably not be stopped by any parental or medical action.

DISCUSSION AND CONCLUSION

We believe that there are instances when a physician should honor an adolescent patient's wish to die. Until the courts, hospitals, and medical societies take a stand on the issue of passive, voluntary euthanasia, the decision is left to the physician. Many considerations must be brought to bear on each case, and the use of a team of consulting specialists, including colleagues in pediatrics, psychiatry, theology, and the law, is optimal. Whether the ultimate responsibility for the decision to allow passive euthanasia should rest with the responsible physician or be diffused onto a small team is a question that warrants much further debate.

As when approaching any dying patient, it is wise to arrive unencumbered with formulas for the occasion, since it will not be covered by rote.[40] It must first be determined whether or not the child has made his decision in a rational and informed manner. Such a decision cannot be obtained in the presence of definable mental illness or persuading outside pressures. The child's cognitive ability to understand death must also be assessed. This ability would be unusual before age 14 or 15. From the physician's personal point of view, he will undoubtedly be influenced by the amount of the child's suffering, the likelihood of improvement in the quality of life now judged unsatisfactory, the closeness of death, the extent of his participation in "causing" the death, as well as his philosophy regarding the dignity of life and the importance of quality and length of life.

The purpose of this chapter is to draw attention to the dilemma of the medical team and the individual physician who are caring for an adolescent who chooses to die. We have outlined the general areas that we think must be considered in each case. Perhaps uniform criteria to weigh these considerations are not sensible at this time, but a body of medical literature on individual cases would be helpful by providing precedents which could be studied and debated. Karen's case was the stimulant for this chapter, and the need for further thought in this area remains our most compelling conclusion.

REFERENCES

1. Freeman JM: Is there a right to die—quickly? J Pediatr **80:**904, 1972.
2. Cooke RE: Whose suffering? J Pediatr **80:**906, 1972.
3. Nelson WE: Editorial comment. J Pediatr **80:**907, 1972.
4. Schowalter JE: Death and the pediatric house officer. J Pediatr **76:**706, 1970.
5. Freud S (1915): Thoughts for the times on war and death. *In* Strachey J (ed): Standard Edition, vol. 14. London, Hogarth Press, 1957, pp 273–288.
6. Inhelder B, Piaget J: The Growth of Logical Thinking. New York, Basic Books, 1958, pp 334–350.
7. Nagy MH: The child's theories concerning death. J Genet Psychol **73:**3, 1948.
8. Solnit AJ, Green M: The pediatric management of the dying child: Part II. The child's reaction to the fear of dying. *In* Solnit AJ, Provence S (eds): Modern Perspectives in Child Development. New York, International Universities Press, 1963, pp 217–228.
9. Feifel H: Death. *In* Farberow NL (ed): Taboo Topics. New York, Atherton Press, 1963, pp 8–21.
10. Hinton JM: Facing death. J Psychosom Res **10:**22, 1966.
11. Kram C, Caldwell JM: The dying patient. Psychosomatics, **10:**293, 1969.
12. Livingston PB, Zimet CN: Death anxiety, authoritarianism and choice of specialty in medical students. J Nerv Ment Dis **140:**222, 1965.

13. O'Connell W, Covert C: Death attitudes and humor appreciation among medical students. Existent Psychiat **6**:433, 1967–68.
14. Lustman SL, Richmond JB: On the acceptance of realistic goals in medicine. *In* Solnit AJ, Provence S (eds:) Modern Perspectives in Child Development. New York, International Universities Press, 1963, pp 558–574.
15. Kasper AM: The doctor and death. *In* Feifel H (ed): The Meaning of Death. New York, McGraw-Hill, 1965, pp 259–270.
16. McKegney FP, Lange P: The decision to no longer live on chronic hemodialysis. Am J Psychiat **128**:267, 1971.
17. De-Nour AK, Czaczkes JW: Emotional problems and reactions of the medical team in a chronic hemodialysis unit. Lancet **2**:987, 1968.
18. Beard BH: Fear of death and fear of life: The dilemma in chronic renal failure, hemodialysis and kidney transplantation. Arch Gen Psychiat **21**:373, 1969.
19. Norton CE: Attitudes toward living and dying in patients on chronic hemodialysis. Ann NY Acad Sci **164**:720, 1969.
20. Abram HS, Moore GL, Westervelt FG: Suicidal behavior in chronic dialysis patients. Am J Psychiat **127**:1199, 1971.
21. Salisbury RE: Behavioral responses of a nine-year-old child on chronic dialysis. J Am Acad Child Psychiat **7**:282, 1968.
22. Mutter AZ: Discussion of Dr. Salisbury's paper. J Am Acad Child Psychiat **7**:290, 1968.
23. Reinhart JB: The doctor's dilemma: Whether or not to recommend continuous renal dialysis or renal hemotransplantation for the child with end-stage renal disease. J Pediatr **77**:505, 1970.
24. Fletcher J: Elective death. *In* Torrey EF (ed): Ethical Issues in Medicine. Boston, Little, Brown & Co. 1968, pp 141–157.
25. Fletcher J: The patient's right to die. *In* Sanders MK (ed): The Crisis in American Medicine. New York, Harper & Row, 1961, pp 128–137.
26. Williams RH: Our role in the generation, modification and termination of life. Arch Intern Med. **124**:215, 1969.
27. Brown NK, Bulger RJ, Laws EH, Thompson DJ: The preservation of life. JAMA **211**:76, 1970.
28. Morison RS: Death: process or event. Science **173**:694, 1971.
29. Kass LR: Death as an event: A commentary on Robert Morison. Science **173**: 698, 1971.
30. Fielding H: Amelia. London, Bell, 1889.
31. Sophocles: Electra. *In* Grene D, Lattimore R (eds): Sophocles II. Chicago, University of Chicago Press, 1957.
32. Holton G: Percy Williams Bridgman. Bull At Scie **18**:22, 1962.
33. Pius XII: The prolongation of life. Pope Speaks **4**:393, 1958.
34. Kelly G: Medico-Moral Programs. St. Louis, The Catholic Hospital Association, 1958, p 135.
35. Gustafson J: Mongolism, parental desires and the right to life. Unpublished. Presented at the International Symposium on Human Rights, Retardation and Research, Washington, DC, October 16, 1971.
36. Responsibility in Investigations on Human Subjects. Medical Research Council, Great Britain, 1963.
37. Curran WJ, Beecher HK: Experimentation in children. A reexamination of legal ethical principles. JAMA **210**:77, 1969.
38. Ramsey P: The Patient as Person. New Haven, Yale University Press, 1970.
39. Morse HN: Legal implications of clinical investigations. Vanderbilt Law Review **20**:747, 1967.
40. Aring CD: Intimations of mortality: In appreciation of death and dying. Ann Intern Med **69**:137, 1968.

Tomas J. Silber, M.D.

6

ABORTION IN ADOLESCENCE: A BIOETHICAL PERSPECTIVE

BIOETHICAL REFLECTION ON ABORTION

Ethical reflection on abortion has been going on for ages and has acquired particular sophistication in this century. (Abortion of course forms part of an even larger debate on what is good and what is right.) For this presentation, I limit myself to reviewing some philosophic contributions of the 1970s. They have been selected because they are representative of diverse contemporary currents of thought, because they are clear, because they are well recognized in their field, and because they have not found their way into the medical and psychosocial literature. I recognize the limitation of reducing a review to concepts worked out in the past few years, but I justify this by the fact that their language is more familiar to our "modern" mind and to the fact that those works *do* incorporate the substantial elements of centuries of reflection on abortion.

The order of publication is followed.

John T. Noonan (1970) considers the morality of abortion from the historical religious tradition.[1] He sees as a crucial point the determination of the humanity of a being; that is, if the fetus is human, it deserves love. Since the religious perspective emphasizes the love of humanity, and since

Reprinted by courtesy of Journal of Current Adolescent Medicine, March 1980.

destruction is the most unloving act, abortion is wrong. Noonan insists on the question of deciding at what point an organism becomes human and is therefore entitled to love. He is concerned with finding some objectively identifiable criterion from which a distinction can be made between human and nonhuman life. Noonan states his conclusion in biologic terms: Whatever is conceived from human parents is human from the moment of conception and therefore entitled to human rights. Certainly in first instance is the right to life. Noonan's philosophy may be thus synthesized: A fetus has full moral status.

Judith Jarvis Thomson (1971) attempts to settle the question of whether abortion is immoral *apart* from the question of whether or not the fetus has full moral status (personhood).[2] Her position is that the rights of the pregnant woman have been completely left out in the considerations of the abortion dilemma. She insists that determining what rights a fetus possesses is but *one* step in determining the moral status of abortion. The *final* step would be to find a just solution to the conflict between the fetal rights and the rights of the woman who is unwillingly pregnant. Thomson states that a woman has a right to an abortion regardless of what rights the fetus has. She illustrates this with the now classic "analogy of the violinist." (Picture yourself waking up one day in bed with a famous violinist. Imagine that your bloodstream has been hooked up to that of the violinist, who happens to have a condition that is certainly going to kill him, unless he is permitted to share your body for a period of nine months. No one else can do it. He will be unconscious all the time and you will have to stay with him, but after the nine months are over he may be unplugged, completely cured.) The question the analogy raises is: What are one's obligations under this circumstance? Her answer is that it would be commendable to save the violinist . . . but it would be incorrect to say that refusal to do so would be murder. The violinist's right to life "does not obligate you to keep him alive."

Michael Tooley (1972) looks for a criterion to determine the right to life. He concludes that although it is true that the fetus is human, this biologic feature has no *moral* significance.[3] Instead, being "*a person*" rather than being genetically human is what determines the right to life. He argues that a right to life appears only when one has the capacity to desire to continue existing "as a subject of experience and other mental states." According to this interpretation, a human being may be eliminated until some time after birth when self-awareness develops. Tooley's philosophy may be thus synthesized: A fetus (and/or newborn) has no moral status.

H. Tristram Engelhardt (1973) analyzes personhood in a way reminiscent of Tooley.[4] But he justifies this by constructing a theory that accounts for the development of varying levels of significance associated with human life. The determining value, he claims, is that of social role. He sees the acquisition of rights as occurring by virtue of our membership in a social context. Infants do relate to persons and evoke responses; therefore, they are entitled to protection. Fetuses cannot play a social role, and therefore abortion is permissible until the moment of viability.

Baruch Brody (1974) rejects the idea that fetal humanity can be resolved on the basis of human definitions or decision.[5] Instead, he considers that this decision can be made based on objective data. Brody does not accept that the crucial objective factors have to do with the genetic code or probability of development. He states that such an objective factor has to do with the "essence of humanity." By that, Brody means what is lost when a human no longer exists.

Brody considers that the criterion for absent life is the nonfunctioning central nervous system, and he argues next "that the fetus becomes a living human being when it acquires that characteristic which is such that its loss entails that a living human being no longer exists." Thus he claims that the fetus is a human being from about six weeks' gestation, the time at which fetal brain activity starts to be noticeable. Brody's philosophy can be expressed as saying that the fetus has no significant moral status during the initial stages of growth but that he *does* have significant moral status beginning at some later stage. John Badertscher (1976) interprets the conflicting positions on abortion as grounded in two different moral orientations, which he describes as liberal and conservative.[6]

The liberal orientation understands freedom as autonomy and therefore claims that giving birth, like other human acts, should be freely chosen. The conservative orientation is based on a different concept of freedom; the freedom of the fetus has to be considered in any decision on abortion. It becomes easy to understand the mutual criticism. The liberal views the conservative as fatalistic and insensitive to the pregnant woman, and the conservative sees the liberal as exalting the power of the individual and excluding the defenseless fetus from any protection. Badertscher insists that the abortion debate has a religious (orientation) dimension and that therefore it is necessary for both positions to "begin to incorporate the deepest concerns of the other side into their own position." He concludes that as a result, the liberal could be led to consider whether the cause of freedom could not be advanced by protection of fetal life while the conservative could be pressed to take account of the real problems of pregnant women.

It is possible to continue with the numerous and insightful views that physicians, ethicists, and theologians have written on the subject. But since the purpose of the review was to set up the background for the discussion of abortion in adolescence, the preceding will suffice.

ABORTION IN ADOLESCENCE: ETHICAL ASPECTS

There is no comparable literature to consider the special situation of the pregnant adolescent. For that reason, I shall attempt to develop some central themes. First of all, I will remark on some peculiar characteristics of adolescents:

- Adolescents are in the midst of a development stage. (This includes cognitive and moral development.)
- Adolescents share with adults the right to privacy.
- Adolescents aim to exercise autonomy.
- The adolescent shares with the child a rather large potential of different outcome and a certain limitation in the understanding of the possible consequence of her actions. (Though not of such a magnitude as to render obsolete the "mature minor" doctrine, this limitation is sufficient to question the degree of responsibility.)

Next, I would like to emphasize a peculiarity of adolescent pregnancy. In spite of its adverse consequences, it still remains a fact that it is a landmark in the girl's life which (especially if carried to term) differentiates her from her nonpregnant peers. This means that she has crossed an ontologic threshold into biologic motherhood. No matter how horrible the circumstances surrounding this, it remains phenomenologically a significant (though often thwarted) biographic event.

Having presented these basic thoughts, I suggest that in the case of an adolescent pregnancy, the moral dilemma of abortion is accentuated by the fact that we are dealing with *two* developing individuals claiming protection. I consider that we have obligations to *both minors*. (This perception refers directly to my visceral understanding of the problem as a pediatrician.)

Another consideration is that the abortion dilemma confronts a morally developing being. This means that in addition to the personal decision of the moment, this will also have a considerable impact on the future and further adolescent moral development.

The time has come to tie all the preceding discussion together. Since the task is ethical reasoning, I shall do this following with the first person singular. This is needed, of course, in order to claim responsibility and in order to generate discussion and future contributions.

I believe abortion is killing. Arguments that the fetus has no moral status or that the fetus acquires this status at a particular stage of gestation violates biologic reality (here I agree with Noonan.) I also believe it is immoral to bring an unwanted child into the world.

The reality of abortion as killing should not remove abortion as an alternative; killing in self-defense may be permissible. It merely means that we should face up to the reality of what the decision to abort entails. My observations in office practice have shown me that the ethical question of abortion is the major source of conflict for the adolescent deciding whether or not to abort. (Their intuitions are indeed of great significance!)

If the adolescent has chosen abortion, the question may be raised: What is the moral significance of the act? It has been variously seen as morally indifferent, as murder, as wrongdoing, as the lesser evil. In addition, I would like to contribute two concepts to further illuminate moral aspects of abortion in adolescence: The concept of "incomplete responsibility" and the "sacrificial" viewpoint.

By "incomplete responsibility," I mean the fact that in many instances the adolescent girl does not have a full understanding of the nature and long-range implications of sexual interactions. (The intuitive perception of this fact is probably the reason subjacent to the "statutory rape" legislation.) Returning to Thomson's analogy: The violinist has been attached without any good previous agreement.

Inasmuch as responsibility relates to morality, there is indeed a difference, in many instances, between adolescent and adult abortion.

By a "sacrificial" viewpoint, I suggest that abortion in adolescence is not an indifferent moral matter and certainly not murder. Instead, I view it as a painful offering made toward the avoidance of future suffering.

Relating to this, I do see the imperative for the adolescent girl not to repeat her abortion. The sacrifice of the fetus should be followed by a compromise (abstinence, contraception, responsible sex, family planning). From this viewpoint, a second abortion should be considered unethical when this implies betrayal of the assumed compromise. This view of mine *does not* imply of course that second abortions should not be allowed. This brings us into the issue of compulsion.

Everything said so far pertains to free ethical discourse. It is inadmissible to force an adolescent to a compulsory abortion and, conversely, to stop her from having an abortion she desires. It is equally immoral to demand that a physician or nurse should participate in an abortion procedure against their will. Even if adolescents have a right, this does not imply a right to force others to perform such an act. (The ethical significance of abortion in adolescence on society in general is beyond the scope of this chapter.)

SUMMARY AND CONCLUSIONS

In the developing adolescent, abortion presents a special dilemma since it affects "two minors."

The ethical question is usually a major source of conflict for the adolescent deciding whether or not to abort.

The principle of autonomy may be a primary guide to deal with adolescent abortion. The issue of incomplete responsibility and the sacrificial viewpoint also deserve consideration.

Although the adolescent and her decision merit our respect and support, neither individual adolescents nor society should view abortion as a policy to be encouraged at the expense of contraception and adoption.

REFERENCES

1. Noonan JT Jr: An almost absolute value in history. *In* Noonan JR Jr (ed): The Morality of Abortion: Legal and Historical Perspectives. Cambridge, Mass, Harvard University Press, 1970.
2. Thomson JJ: In defense of abortion. Philos Public Affairs 1:4766, 1971.

3. Tooley M: Abortion and infanticide. Philos Public Affairs 1:37, 1972.
4. Engelhardt HT: The ontology of abortion. Ethics 84:217, 1974.
5. Brody B: On the humanity of the fetus. *In* Perkins RL (ed): Abortion: Pro and Con. Cambridge, Mass, Sheakman Publishing Co, 1974.
6. Bradertscher J: Religious dimensions of the abortion debate. Studies in Religion 6(2):177, 1976–1977.

SECTION TWO FURTHER READINGS

1. Abrams N, Buckner MD (eds): Medical Ethics, Bradford Books. Cambridge, MA, The MIT Press, 1983.
2. Jonsen AR, Siegler M, Winslade WJ: Clinical Ethics. New York, McMillan Publishing Co., Inc., 1982.
3. Kuhse H: Debate: Extraordinary Means and the Sanctity of Life. J Med Ethics 7:74–82, 1981.
4. President's Commission for the Study of Ethical Problems in Medicine and Behavioral Research: Deciding to Forego Life-Sustaining Treatment, A Report on the Ethical, Medical and Legal Issues in Treatment Decisions. Washington, DC, US Government, 1983.
5. Rachels J: Active and Passive Euthanasia. N Engl J Med 292:78, 1978.
6. Silber T: Parental Consent to Euthanasia. The Hastings Center Report, 10:26, 1980.
7. Silber T: Abortion in Adolescence: The Ethical Dimension. Adolescence, 15:462–474, 1980.

SECTION THREE

PROFESSIONAL/PATIENT RELATIONSHIP

This section deals with the general issue of the moral obligation of the pediatrician to his patients. It is initiated by Sanford Leikin, who scrutinizes one particular issue: truth-telling and deception in the care of the pediatric patient. He deals with the subject of paternalism and exposes the ethical and psychologic elements concerning nondisclosure as it relates to the autonomy of a minor.

A profound account of the nature of ethical development is given by Joseph Noshpitz. It is based on observations and reflections made during his many years of dedication to child development and psychoanalytic theory. It has been specially written for this anthology because it is important that the pediatrician become acquainted with the fascinating process of moral development during childhood. Understanding the ethics of childhood can indeed enhance pediatrician-patient communication. This section concludes with Silber's analysis of the ethical dimension in the relationship between the doctor and his adolescent patients.

Sanford L. Leikin, M.D.

7

AN ETHICAL ISSUE IN PEDIATRIC CANCER CARE: NONDISCLOSURE OF A FATAL PROGNOSIS

Case report: A 13-year-old boy was diagnosed as having lymphatic cancer in February 1980. The diagnosis was first presented to the parents. The physician stated that the prognosis was poor because of the advanced nature of the disease and suggested that the patient be told about his disease and its prognosis. The parents agreed to have the physician tell the boy about his disease and its treatment but not about the poor prognosis, to which the physician acquiesced.

When the discussion was held with the patient, he asked only questions concerning his capability to return to participation in sports; a guarded statement concerning this was given. He was treated and responded well initially but then relapsed, and his treatment was changed. Several conferences were held with the parents during this time, and the poor prognosis of this condition was reiterated. They continued to have difficulty accepting this.

When the second treatment failed, the physician told the parents that no other conventional treatment was available but that experimental drugs could be tried or that palliative treatment could be given at home. The parents were again encouraged to inform the boy of his poor prognosis, but again they resisted that suggestion. During a discussion with the patient

Reprinted by courtesy of Pediatric Annals 10:37, 1981.

about his treatment, however, the patient asked what had been told to his parents that had not been told to him about his illness. The doctor told him that his prognosis was poor and what treatment options were available. He refused the experimental drug treatment and accepted the home-care program. He died in November.

The general issue that surrounds this case is that of truth-telling and deception in pediatric cancer care. Other issues are paternalism and the autonomy of the minor. In this chapter, I discuss these issues from psychologic and ethical points of view and try to show how their emphases change with time or during the course of an illness.

TRUTH TELLING AND VERACITY

The major early medical oaths and codes were silent on the subject of what physicians should tell patients. Mention is made of confidentiality but there is no reference to honesty toward patients. The Code of Ethics of the American Medical Association of 1847 even endorsed some forms of deception by stating that the physician had a sacred duty "to avoid all things which have a tendency to discourage the patient and to depress his spirits."

Recently, however, there has been a revision in that approach, and the second principle adopted by the A.M.A. House of Delegates at its 1980 annual meeting states that "a physician shall deal honestly with patients and colleagues, and strive to expose those physicians deficient in character or competence, or who engage in fraud or deception."

Bok has described the discomfort of physicians that can occur when they talk to patients about their illness.[1] "Physicians, moreover, are acutely aware of the uncertainties of diagnosis and prognosis," she notes. "They know how hard it is to give meaningful and correct answers to questions regarding health and illness. They also know that disclosing their uncertainty or their pessimistic prognosis can reduce those benefits which depend on faith and the placebo effect. They dislike being the bearers of uncertain or bad news as much as anyone else. Sitting down to discuss an illness with a patient truthfully and sensitively may take much-needed time away from other patients. For all these reasons, physicians and other health care professionals often prefer not to be bound by codes or rules that might limit their ability to suppress, delay, and even distort the information about their patients' conditions."

Patients, as consumers, have become increasingly aware of their right to be adequately informed, and recently the Patient's Bill of Rights, published by the American Hospital Association, stated that the patient has the right to receive information concerning his diagnosis, treatment, and prognosis, except when not medically advisable, in which case the information should be made available to an appropriate person in his behalf.[2]

Philosophers and religious thinkers have debated issues dealing with deception and truth-telling. They have generally regarded truthfulness as fundamental to the existence of trust among human beings, and therefore, as an indispensable trait for persons to strive for. They have, however, been divided into those who, like Kant, believed that there can be no sufficient justification for lying, and those who believed that there are times when deception can be justifiably undertaken.[3] Kant stated that lies are morally reprehensible whether or not they harm others, since they rest on immoral maxims (general rules) and degrade the liar himself. Bentham disagreed.[4] He argued that if a falsehood were uttered that had no harmful effect, it could not possibly constitute an offense either to others or to the liar. Thus, for Bentham, consequences determine the moral acceptability of a lie, whereas this is not so in Kant's philosophy. The utilitarian position in moral philosophy, expounded by Bentham, was elaborated and defended by Sidgwick, who took for granted that certain lies, such as those sometimes told to invalids and children, are necessary and could be warranted by being in the best interests of those thus deceived.[5] But this process of weighing gains and losses, advocated by utilitarians, runs into great problems in actual application. It is hard enough to make such estimates for one person; but to make them for several, as must be done in all cases of deception (which are, by definition, interpersonal) is well nigh impossible except in the simplest of cases.

Three arguments for the duty of veracity are particularly applicable to the relationship between health-care professionals and patients.[6] The first holds that the duty of veracity is part of the respect we owe to persons. Within biomedical contexts, respect for persons is commonly expressed through the principle of autonomy. Not to solicit consent for treatment from patients is to violate their autonomy and to fail to respect them as persons. Consent, however, cannot express autonomy unless it is informed, and it therefore depends on communication and ultimately on truth-telling. Second, some philosophers argue that the duty of veracity is an expression of the duty of fidelity or promise-keeping. When we communicate with others by language, we implicitly promise that we will not deceive our listeners as to the facts or our opinions. By entering into a relationship in the context of therapy, the patient not only retains a general right to the truth but gains a special right to the truth regarding diagnosis, prognosis, procedures, etc. Third, relationships of trust between human beings are necessary for fruitful interaction and cooperation; such cooperation depends on persons' confidence that they can rely upon others to respect the principle of veracity. Lying undermines the relationship of trust and produces undesirable consequences. The liar thus fails to show respect for other persons and their autonomy, violates implicit contracts, and also threatens relationships based on trust.

The principle of veracity refers to more than lying, which is defined as intentionally deceiving another so as to get the other to believe what is false. One cannot accidentally tell a lie. Veracity also includes broader issues of deception, which encompasses acts other than lying, eg, mere withholding of information. The duty of veracity, broadly construed, requires nondeception, but some acts of nondeception probably do not threaten the relationship of trust, as overt lying does. Both lies and other forms of deception are *prima facie* wrong and stand in need of justification. To this end, several philosophers have shown how one might go beyond the Kantian position (which allows for no moral conflict once truthfulness is at stake) and also beyond the utilitarian position (with its problems of application and its assumption that there is nothing inherently valuable about truthfulness apart from its consequences). Ross, in *The Right and the Good,* argues that there is a *prima facie* duty of fidelity, which includes that of veracity, but that such a duty can conflict with other *prima facie* duties, such as that of "not injuring others," or that of "beneficence." And Warnock, in *The Object of Morality,* similarly stresses the possibility of conflict among duties. He states that the four virtues of nonmaleficence, beneficence, justice, and veracity are required if things are not to go quite so badly among human beings as they otherwise might, given the nature of the human predicament. But there can be no assurance that they will always work together; at times they may even be in such a conflict that no good solution exists.

NONDISCLOSURE

In the previous case report, the form of deception that was used immediately after the diagnosis of this child was nondisclosure about his prognosis. My emphasis in the following pages concerns issues of nondisclosure involving pediatric patients.

Beauchamp and Childress list several arguments for limited nondisclosure of some diagnoses and prognoses in therapeutic settings.[8] The first argument represents what Sidgwick called "benevolent deception."[5] It holds that disclosure of a diagnosis would violate the duties of beneficence and nonmaleficence by causing serious consequences. Cousins, in a recent editorial, extends the idea that providing a grim prognosis can even be self-fulfilling.[9] I believe that this magical thinking does occur in the minds of parents when it is suggested that bad prognoses be provided to their sick child, but, in fact, there is no sound scientific evidence of this consideration.

One objection to disclosure is based on the uncertainty of predicting consequences such as anxiety, depression, and suicide. A perception that individuals have is that there will be a permanent depressing effect on the patient after delivery of a bad prognosis. To hear the pronouncement of a bad prognosis is very frightening and upsetting to all concerned. It is not usually totally overwhelming, however, and many adults and older children may be relieved at hearing a serious prognosis, since it may not be as bad as they imagined. They usually can cope after such information has been presented. For instance, Moore and associates report that although suicide is a common cause of death in adolescence, there were no suicide attempts among 182 adolescents with cancer in a six-year experience.[10] Binger et al also report that there was no evidence during the course of the illness or during their interviews with the family after death that those children who were told that they had leukemia had greater difficulty in coping than did their counterparts to whom nothing had been said directly.[11] Karon has pointed out that teenagers gain emotional strength from the knowledge that there are ways of treating their disease even though the likelihood of success may be low.[12] Teenagers use denial as one of the major defense mechanisms against cancer. The child shuts the prognosis out of his mind, and continues to hope that he will get well, even in the face of obvious setbacks.

The more telling objections to "benevolent deception" stress violations of the principles of respect for persons and fidelity, as well as the long-term threat to the relationship of trust between physicians and patients. This is exceedingly poignant in pediatric cancer care, since it is recognized that many fatally ill children as young as five years of age sense that they are dying even when not informed, and that the frequency begins to rise at about age six to reach almost 100% in late adolescence.[13] If this is the case, nondisclosure seriously interferes with the physician's key role in managing children, in which they can have a trusting relationship with him, and can feel free to discuss their concerns and get honest answers.

A second argument for nondisclosure and deception is that health-care professionals cannot know or cannot communicate the "whole truth," and if they could, many patients would not be able to comprehend and understand it. This is obviously of great concern in managing children because of their limited ability to conceptualize the prognostic implication of a fatal illness. Our understanding is based on our knowledge of children's emotional reactions to death and dying—an understanding that has been reviewed extensively by Schowalter and Easson.[13,14] Schowalter divides children's attitudes about and conceptualizations of death into four developmental periods: the infant and toddler period (first three years of life), the preschool period (ages three to six), the latency age period (seven to ten), and the preadolescent and adolescent period. Obviously these attitudes and concepts do not change abruptly at a given age but evolve gradually and with wide individual variation.

Death is not yet a familiar or realistic concept for the child younger than the age of three, but the fear of separation from protecting, comforting objects is present in its most terrifying intensity. Sometime between the ages of three and five most children first comprehend the fact of death as something that happens to others. The concept of death remains relatively unstable in children of this age group, and they cannot comprehend its permanency. In addition, they have no real idea of the meaning of time or of the future. The dying child of this age no longer responds purely with separation anxiety but often feels his illness is a retribution for bad thoughts or actions. During the early school-age period, the permanency and universality of death gradually, though incompletely, make their impact on the child. Studies by Piaget show that children of this age group attribute death to an external agent which causes the organism to die or cease to move.[15] It seems that the fear of death per se first makes its appearance at this time, and that the child is horrified, confused, and angered. A feeling of responsibility for the illness remains strong at this age. When a parental person, like a doctor or a nurse, tells a seven-year-old child that he will die in three months, the boy is likely to see this statement as an absolute decision; he may wait for fate to strike him down exactly three months hence. He watches the calendar and marks off each day in his mind. Anxiety about the meaning of the specific prognosis may so drain this child emotionally and physically that he becomes much less able to face or to cope with his illness than otherwise would be the case.

As Schowalter has noted, the universality and permanence of death finally become comprehensible to a child at about the age of 10 or 11.[13] When he reaches this age, he has an almost-adult capacity to understand death, and so his response to being told of his own terminal illness will be more like that of an adult. Because of his illness, the child of this age is faced with regression, loss of control, and the need for external help.

The third argument for nondisclosure and deception is that some patients, particularly the sick and dying, do not really want to know the truth about their condition. Some children who are dying do not want to be told. Schowalter recounts how an adolescent explained it, "If you tell me I'm dying, it's a fact; but if only I think it, I can believe it or not depending on how I feel that day." We know that during the latency period (six to ten or eleven years of age) some children begin to ask if they are dying. However, they seldom really want to know the truth, but are expressing their realization that they are very sick. Most children are content with an explanation of *why* they are feeling so bad with reassurance that they will be taken care of.[13]

Some children, either explicitly or by other means, indicate that they do not want to be informed of the prognosis. Bluebond-Langner describes the coping mechanism of "mutual pretense" that leukemia children practiced along with parents and staff because it offered each of them a way to fulfill the roles and responsibilities necessary for maintaining membership in society in the face of that which threatened the fulfillment of social obligations and continued membership.[17] Some would argue that the patient has a *duty* to seek the truth, not merely a right to the truth; to force unwanted information, however, is to act paternalistically and to violate the patient's autonomy. There are other considerations relating to this issue which will be dealt with later.

PARENTAL RESPONSIBILITIES AND RIGHTS IN NONDISCLOSURE

Parental and family considerations may play a role in nondisclosure of a fatal prognosis to adults and children but are stronger in relation to children whose limited conceptual capacity and autonomy are more clearly recognized. In the case report at the beginning of this chapter, the parents insisted on nondisclosure. What ethical considerations might influence physicians and others to follow that mandate? At the time of diagnosis the parents are better acquainted with the child, which could be an important source (and maybe the only source) of information for the physician concerning the child's level of maturity, his views about life and illness, and the choices he might make.

A more telling argument is that physicians have a moral duty not to interfere with the child's dependent relationship with the parents. As Ackerman has stated, "a sick child who is victimized by a catastrophic disease such as childhood cancer is very much preoccupied in coming to emotional terms with that disease and all that it involves. There is adjustment to the unusual hospital surroundings, invasive procedures, pain, and his own state of fear. In dealing with his own state of mind, a child depends very much on his family's assistance."[18] The parents possess the relationship, resources, and expertise to render aid to support the child under these circumstances. They can provide physical and financial support, solace, and moral and religious guidance. Since it will be the parents to a great extent who will provide most of the emotional comfort and guidance to the child, they need to agree to disclosure so that they can be prepared for its consequences. If they do not accept and are not emotionally prepared for dealing with the disclosure themselves, the child's ability to handle the situation may be adversely affected.

Interwoven with these parental considerations, and difficult to differentiate from them, is the distress parents may feel when the child is told of his fatal prognosis—an act that in itself could be taken as distressing to the child. But although this may initially be disturbing to the child, as mentioned previously there do not appear to be any long-term deleterious emotional or physical effects when such a disclosure is made. It is also the parents' autonomy that is being interfered with, however, when their insistence on nondisclosure is not honored.

The danger, if we speak of parental rights instead of parental duties and responsibilities, is that the confusion of the "my child" of ownership is likely to be aggravated. This means that the parents are held morally responsible for those things that result from their actions and they can be praised or blamed on account of the consequences. This is, indeed, one way of establishing a link between causal responsibility and moral responsibility. If a parent abuses a child and the child is injured, we hold the parent responsible for that injury, since the injury was the result of the parent's actions. What is needed to establish a responsibility, not to mention a right, is a different matter when the child is sick, however. In the child-abuse case the parent is responsible for the effect, which is the child's injury; likewise, in the case of procreation the parents are responsible for the effect, which is the child. Moral obligations to others are not grounded only in this kind of causal connection, they arise simply because people are people. Essentially, what is being stated is that health-care providers also have expertise in the care of sick children. Under these circumstances, the parents are not the only ones who are morally responsible. Since the health-care provider knows that the older child with a terminal illness realizes its seriousness and probable fatality, it is the provider's moral obligation to establish a meaningful communication with the patient, to discuss the illness and its prognosis, and thus relieve his feelings of fear, anxiety, and sense of helplessness and loneliness.

Because both the parents and physicians have their own intrinsic needs and attitudes that might interfere, there is no guarantee that any one such person exists who can make the "morally correct decision" for the sick child, as Langham points out.[19] All that can be suggested is a system of checks and balances.

AUTONOMY AND PATERNALISM

According to Beauchamp and Childress, autonomy is a form of personal liberty of action where the individual determines his or her own course of action in accordance with a plan chosen by himself or herself.[20] The autonomous person is one who not only deliberates about and chooses such plans, but also is capable of acting on the basis of such deliberations, just as a truly independent government has autonomous control of its territories and policies. A person's autonomy is his or her independence, self-reliance, and self-contained ability to decide. A person of diminished autonomy, by contrast, is highly dependent on others and, in at least some respect, incapable of deliberating or acting on the basis of such deliberations.

The term *autonomy* is thus quite broad, for it can refer to both the will and action in society; and internal and external constraint on action can limit it. When the patient described at the beginning of the chapter requested to know what had been told to his parents that had not been told to him, he indicated that he wished to exert his autonomy. What caused him to ask that question at that time we do not know but only can conjecture. It may have been the passage of time from diagnosis, which allowed a developmental process to occur. For example, children between the ages of 11 and 15 were found to be more conforming to pressures from others than were children between the ages of seven and nine.[21] Thus the older child may be less assertive in seeking knowledge about his or her illness. He may also have asked the question because of a growing realization that his condition was worsening, since he had had more pain following his initial relapse. Or it could be that he no longer felt that he could depend on his parents to provide the information that he needed. It could also have been a combination of these internal factors. In any event, the weights of the various ethical issues had now changed. As stated previously, external factors are involved in autonomy. In the case of this patient, it was the recognition by the physician of the patient's wish to know more about his condition that led him to respond by disclosing the prognosis.

The physician could thus support the patient by providing information to him about the course of his disease and its treatment and discussing his concerns with him. The fact that the patient requested information about the prognosis of his disease is critical to this discussion. By this request the patient declared his independence from his parents in seeking and receiving information about this aspect of his illness, and thus asserted his individuality. But more important, this boy, who said he wanted to be informed, claimed a justifiable right.

A fundamental element of autonomy is the recognition of competence to comprehend the significance of imparted information—in this case the actuality of his fatality. Freud stated that no one can ever fully comprehend his own death; however, as previously mentioned, the grasping of possibilities and limitations of one's self in relation to a definite future do develop during adolescence.[22] Further, I believe that this minor's request for further information about his prognosis indicated the awareness of the possibility of his poor prognosis. Whether or not the latter is the case, the claim for candor that he has made takes first precedence in this situation, and the burden of proof should fall to those who judge that this claim should be denied. It must be kept in mind that the cognitive understanding of death can exist without the emotional maturity necessary to make a final decision regarding one's own life, but the just recognition of this minor's right to be informed and the response to it with candor and a reduction of paternalistic overprotection is his first step (and maybe his last) toward autonomy.

In this chapter I have tried to expose the ethical and psychologic elements concerning nondisclosure as it related to the autonomy of a minor. Truth-telling remains one of the greatest challenges of pediatric oncology, and we must continue to probe children's, parents', and health-care providers' minds for clues to help resolve this dilemma. In the meanwhile, as Schowalter states, "What is most important is that there be an atmosphere of openness that allows the patient to ask as much or as little as he wishes. The more painful a decision is, the more we wish to establish a rule to cover it: it would be much easier if there were an age, type of diagnosis, family circumstance, or other indicator that could be relied on to determine correctly what to tell the child. The only true indicator, however, is the child and the only measurement is the caregiver's sensitivity" and, I would add, the parents' as well.[16]

With these caveats concerning developmental limitations, and the recognition of the possible presence of the coping mechanism of "mutual pretense," health-care providers need to search for changes in the psychologic state of the patient and parents so that as complete disclosure as possible can be provided during illness.

REFERENCES

1. Bok S: Truth-telling, II. Ethical aspects. *In* Reich WT (ed): Encyclopedia of Bioethics. New York, Macmillan Publishing Company, 1978, p 1683.

2. American Hospital Association: A Patient's Bill of Rights. Chicago, American Hospital Association, 1972.
3. Quoted in Bok. supra, p 1685.
4. Bentham J: An introduction to the principles of morals and legislation. *In* The English Philosophy from Bacon to Mill, New York, Modern Library, 1939, p 791 ff.
5. Quoted in Beauchamp T and Childress J: Principles of Biomedical Ethics. New York, Oxford University Press, 1979, p 205.
6. Beauchamp T, Childress J: supra, p 202.
7. Bok S: supra, p 1686.
8. Beauchamp T, Childress J: supra, p 205.
9. Cousins NA: A layman looks at truth-telling in medicine. JAMA 244: 1929–1930, 1980.
10. Moore C, Holton C, Marten, G: Psychologic problems in the management of adolescents and malignancy. Clin. Pediatr. 8: 464–473, 1969.
11. Binger C et al: Childhood leukemia. Emotional impact on patient and family. N Engl J Med 280: 414–418, 1969.
12. Karon M: The physician and the adolescent with cancer. Pediatr. Clin. North Am. 20: 965–973, 1973.
13. Schowalter J: The child's reaction to his own terminal illness. *In* Schoenberg B, Carr AC, Peretz, D, Kutscher AH (eds): Loss and Grief: Psychological Management in Medical Practice. New York, Columbia University Press, 1970.
14. Easson W: The Dying Child. Springfield, Ill., Charles C Thomas, 1977.
15. Piaget J: The Child's Conception of the World. New York, The Humanities Press, 1929.
16. Schowalter J: The reactions of caregivers dealing with fatally ill children and their families. *In* Sahler OJZ: The Child and Death. St. Louis, C. V. Mosby Company, 1978.
17. Bluebond-Langner M: The Private Worlds of Dying Children. Princeton, NJ, Princeton University Press, 1978.
18. Ackerman T: Fooling ourselves with child autonomy and assent in nontherapeutic clinical research. Clin. Res. 27: 349–358, 1979.
19. Langham P: Parental consent: Its justification and limitations. Clin. Res. 27: 349–358, 1979.
20. Beauchamp T, Childress J: supra. p 5.
21. Costanzo P, Shaw M: Conformity as a function of age level. Child Dev. 37: 967–975, 1966.
22. Freud S: Thoughts for the times on war and death. *In* Strackey J (ed): The Standard Edition of the Complete Psychological Works of Sigmund Freud. Volume 2. London, Hogarth Press, 1958, pp 334–350.

Joseph D. Noshpitz, M.D.

8

UNDERSTANDING THE SCHOOL CHILD'S ETHICS

In classic psychoanalytic theory, the agency of the mind that is the bearer and shaper of all mature ethical development is the superego.[1] It is formed at approximately five to seven years of age, as part of the developmental surge that helps put to rest the child's oedipal strivings. Functionally, it acts to contain, to control, and to inhibit the murderous and incestuous yearnings of that time. Once formed, the superego continues to function thereafter as an integral part of personality.

Structurally, the superego consists of an organization of functions of somewhat diverse character. To start, there are all the limits, the forbiddings, the containments, and the many "no-no's" that have accumulated over time. These are now assembled into this one complex structure to become part of a hierarchy of internalized "lessons," of which we are thereafter aware without knowing how we know them. At the base of this assemblage are the great taboos of our culture. We know that cannibalism, the idea of eating human flesh, disgusts and dismays us; the very thought is unsettling. We know that any suggestion of touching feces, or of smelling them, begets intense aversive reactions—for many of us this extends to all types of messiness and dirt, and even to simple disorder. We know that the idea of torture and gross body injury is dreadful, that we are appalled by accounts of sadism. All this had been built in from very early in our childhood, each as a separate mandate against biting or smearing or hurting. Now, however, all these coalesce. They become part of the superego and fit together with the second great wave of forbiddings, those that derive from the oedipal situation. These have to do with themes like patricide, matricide, incest, and certain aspects of sexual curiosity and exhibitionism. Here are formidable taboos indeed, and as we erect them within ourselves, within the hierarchy that is becoming the superego, we go through one of the greatest steps toward socialization that we are ever fated to take: we give up the vaunting fantasy leaps of the preschool years and settle down to become little boys and little girls. As part of the process, we take into ourselves the values, the mores, the ethics, and the outlooks that our parents have been communicating over the years. We begin to share their mortality and to join their culture. Perhaps of equal importance, we begin—just begin at this point—to share as well in some of their ideals.

In short, this is a time fraught with immense significance for the emergence of a sense of ethics. Prior to superego formation, there are many learned external prohibitions; after it forms, there is an internal organized system of values, inhibitions, and aspirations to challenge and guide behavior, and to regulate self-esteem. It is here that ethics first comes into play.

We have given some thought to superego formation, but it is important to keep in mind that once formed, the superego behaves like any other dimension of personality; it continues to grow and to change over time. Under optimal circumstances, it will show evidence of positive development, which will take it to new heights of richness and maturity. By the same token, however, it will also exhibit the vulnerabilities that are part and parcel of all growth, so that when conditions for healthy progress are adverse, its advance may be arrested, it may regress to yet more primitive levels of function, or it may proceed to develop in a skewed and unhealthy fashion.[2]

Its first major growth phase comes during latency. With the "conquest" of the oedipal impulse, the superego can enter a state of partial quietude. In effect, the demands for its services are less, and its task becomes more one of maintenance of status quo than of active struggle with impulse. In fact, however, there arises a host of new impulses; it proceeds to develop, although in a somewhat different realm and in quite another fashion.

In the latency epoch, the child is relieved of the need to struggle with the consuming oedipal passions of an earlier time. Indeed, during this era, under optimal conditions much of the tension in the parent-child relationship is lessened. Roles and territories become clear: child is child and parent is parent. With this occurrence, the youngsters are far more available for attachments outside the home, and the new realm for development becomes the interpersonal issue of peer engagement. However, this too is experienced as a complex environment with its own hierarchies, its own threats and principles, and its own rewards. At the outset it is a trackless waste, a territory of unbounded possibility. The youngster needs a chart in order to find his or her path. It is precisely this work, the inner organization of a set of guiding principles for the safe threading of one's way through this wilderness of peer interaction, that takes form as the superego of the latency period. This is added on to the body of principles, taboos, and precepts that is already in place. The fact that one has built-in inhibition about incestuous yearnings does little to help answer questions of whose turn it is to play, or who is really the winner in a particular exchange. A new array of orderings is necessary, and it is at this time of life that it comes to be organized.

Much of the latency superego is formed within the context of social group pressures. What emerges is a sort of ethic of latency whose tenets serve principally to regulate the interplay of peers. This moral code prevails chiefly during this time of life; it does not appear earlier, and it is not likely to dominate later. That is to say, it is not likely to do so where development proceeds as it should and the person matures well. In many cases, however, this state of affairs does not ensue. Latency may be the natural time for these tenets to flourish, but many times they persist as the individual's basic ethical stance. They involve such assertions as: "Finders keepers, losers weepers," "first come, first served," "everyone was doing it, so I did it too," "he did it to me first, so I was just getting even."

It seems fair to say that the aforementioned are largely territorial statements, principles built on retention of what one has and revenge for what one has lost. They also speak for the power of the group and its central role in determining what is right and what one may or may not do. It is not surprising that these principles should prevail. Anal regression is very much a part of latency, and it is in the anal phase that social pressure, shaming, and the eyes of the significant other are among the determinative forces at work shaping the child's behavior.[3] It is also then that the critical concept of territoriality seems to be first in evidence. Hence, the ethic of latency is primarily an anal stage ethic, an ethic of boundaries and entitlements, of possession and retention, of pride and retaliation. Dominating it is the basic sense of revenge as a regulating principle in life; it is with revenge rather than with some abstract conception of justice that the youngster feels preoccupied. "Getting even" with someone, getting back at someone, paying them back for what they did to you—these become matters of consuming interest to the latency period child. When an insult is extended, the retort that restores equilibrium is: "You're another." There is a fundamental need to assert and to maintain a balance in human affairs.

As latency proceeds, however, a more general and abstract statement of this position emerges. Above all else, this stance becomes the guiding principle for ethical issues; it sets a basic style for the resolution of conflict. In this instance an element emerges that does persist well into later life for everyone: the main goal to be sought in exchanges with one's peers is fairness. That is to say, the sense of balance, of equal weighting of good, of respect for everyone's boundaries, of equality of entitlements, of evenhandedness in the award of both punishments and plaudits—such general statements as these become the measure of the child's sense of justice and injustice. This pervades the group interactions, but even more important, it applies to the treatment expected from authority figures such as parents, teachers, scout leaders, coaches, policemen, and the like. If a child gets smacked for doing something and now another does the same thing, then he or she should get the same punishment.

The intensity of the emotions generated by such issues is considerable. Children experience the maintenance of this balance as a vital dimension of their well-being; if a parent or teacher shows preferential treatment toward another child, there is a distinct sense of outrage, a feeling of mistreatment, and on some level at least, a yearning to protest. There are many situations where protest is unwise, even unthinkable, yet the child who views things in this light will at least murmur to himself about the unfairness of it all.

Developmentally, the fairness doctrine probably emerges from the sense of narcissistic boundaries and the vulnerability that the child experiences at these sites. In a narcissistic reaction, one feels each invasion and each onslaught as a sort of penetration of one's perimeter. He seeks relief by undoing that, by "paying back" or "getting even." By extension, one must retaliate—take suitable revenge—and only then can the wound to the self be eased. Once there is equivalent damage done, the off-balance feeling is at least to some extent set right, and the sense of disequilibrium is eased. One is no longer troubled by the nagging feeling of bias, of disadvantage, of things being out of kilter. The sense of proportion is restored, the dent in one's sense of integrity is smoothed, and the perimeter is no longer sending back shock waves of pain.

Hence the latency period child becomes very much caught up in this talion principle; "an eye for an eye and a tooth for a tooth" sounds very good to him. In his eyes, this is just; the fair way to do things. Fairness becomes one of the guiding principles of his life. Many such a child spends long hours puzzling over or bemoaning some episode in which he feels he was treated unfairly; indeed, the child may remember this for a long time, in some cases even for a lifetime. More than that, he will not only mourn the dents in his periphery, he will seek redress. He will fight if he can; he will refuse to speak to the offending other; he will be sullen, pout, or avoid the authority figure whom he regards as the cause of the unfair dealings; and he will tend in a host of ways to communicate his sense of outrage. Such motives underlie the common "spiteful" behavior so often seen in such children. Someone else is mistreated just to make him feel bad, eg, someone's toy is broken, his doll disfigured, his homework defaced or torn up, "just for spite." Occasionally, it turns out that the vandal is simply sadistic and acts in this way as part of his pursuit of pleasure. More often, however, that child has experienced a slight or a sense of personal injury on some level, and has found this way to react. In his own view, he may be redressing an imbalance in keeping with some inner equation that demands such a step.

As latency goes on, however, an additional dimension is added to the superego. This also has anal stage derivatives but takes the form of adherence to rules. The two-year-old is forever learning the rules of everything; a good many of the no-no's that are so famous at that time of life are in effect rules in themselves, or the response to the violation of rules that the child has not yet learned. The acquisition of rules is a slow, ongoing process that proceeds all through childhood, but it is in latency that this truly comes into its own. Prior to this, rules were a means to an end; at this point they become an end in themselves. It is now that the rules as such become objects of intense emotional involvement; items to be agreed on and then maintained, defended, and, if necessary, fought over.

What seems to happen is that rules are taken into the individual child's superego, and they become part of his or her personal perimeter. A rule violation within a social context, be it a card game or a ball game, now assumes the stature of a personal slight. The child observes the breach with intense concern and may come rushing in seeking to defend and redress this violation with vociferous energy. The more shy and frightened individual may react with withdrawal, tears, and every evidence of being stricken. A not uncommon reaction is, "if that's the way you're gonna play, I won't play with you anymore." The particular response has to do with the temperament of the child and with his capacity to assert himself in the face of opposition; obviously children will vary widely in this respect. The inner sense of outrage and violation because a rule has been dishonored, however, is probably close to universal.

The ability to abide by rules in itself requires a certain amount of emotional maturity. After all, it is inevitable that if one plays a game, there will be some times when one will lose. And what is the child to do then? In particular, what is the more narcissistically oriented child to do, the one who cannot tolerate frustration, who has a high level of expectation or entitlement? What such a child does characteristically is to change the rules. The superego imperative is a powerful one and not lightly gainsaid; except in the more extreme instances of narcissistic disorder, the matter of rules cannot simply be ignored. The child feels the prick of conscience—rules are important and must be obeyed. The compromise that is available is a simple one: alter the rules so that you always win. Do so each time if necessary, and deform them beyond recognition if you must, but spare yourself the pain of defeat and see to it that you win!

The key variable here is the fact that at least the form of the rule structure is maintained. The child does not challenge the fact that rules are real, present, and important; he works within this framework. It is this regard for rules that is the key; it tells how vital it is to preserve this developmental emergent even in the face of unusual levels of dysfunction.

Here we can perceive a nascent part of superego organization that achieves its greatest growth spurt during latency. Rules do not mean too much to the preschooler; relationship structures are more important then. It is in the grade-school years that games and sports, and, for that matter, manners and rituals begin to emerge as objects of primary importance to the children; they learn these things avidly and feel about them keenly. If they understand the rules, they feel comfort, and if they violate them, the more healthy children feel guilt, or at least a sense of shame. Even if they win, the win is tarnished—they did not "really" win. The reaction is that typical of a superego response. Often, they will feel guilty or let down; sometimes they will confess and seek to undo.

The matter of rules and the previously mentioned issue of fairness tend to converge and to coalesce as latency proceeds. A game is fair if it is played by the rules. If an exception to the rule is made, it's not fair—unless it's agreed that the other fellow, or the other team, can also make the same exception. Then, in effect, there is social agreement that the rule shall be altered and the interaction can proceed.

IMPLICATIONS FOR LATER DEVELOPMENT

It is evident that such an aspect of superego formation is a far cry from the issues of incest and murder, which originally brought this agency of mind into being. By the same token, learning about a violation of rules does not evoke the same reaction as the idea of someone engaging in sex with or physically destroying a parent. Clearly, the emotional impact of the one is not to be compared with that of the other. On the other hand, the matter of rules is a far more ubiquitous part of our everyday lives than is the concern with oedipal issues.

In effect, the latency period superego builds in what one might call the "traffic rules" of life. This is the point in development in which these vital social channels are laid out, when the properties and the regulations are stated that govern the everyday intercourse among people.[4] The issues addressed are by no means trivial; when traffic rules are violated, bad things can happen. However, the majority of such rules and their violations do not have life-and-death implications. They are the petty, everyday annoyances, the inconvenient limitations on the facile expression of impulse and on the assertions of self that make social living possible. Examples are having to wait in line and keeping one's place in line instead of cutting in ahead of others, and striving to advance in one's job by fair means rather than foul.

Perhaps the ultimate expression of this superego level is to be found in such products of human effort as "Robert's Rules of Order"—where each item and nuance of group interaction falls under a rule of some kind so that all expression and communication follow a predetermined sequence of orderings and priorities. The law at this moment in development is to follow rules; it is this development in particular that sets the foundation for what ultimately becomes the rule of law.[5]

REFERENCES

1. Freud S: The Ego and the Id. London, Hogarth Press, 1927.
2. Freud S: The Passing of the Oedipus Complex. *In* Freud S: Collected Papers II. London, Hogarth Press, 1924.
3. Bomstein B: On Latency. *In* Eissle R et al (eds): The Psychoanalytic Study

of the Child, Volume X, New York, International Universities Press, 1951, pp 279–285.
4. Gough JW: The Social Contract. Oxford, The Clarendon Press, 1957.
5. Rawls J: A Theory of Justice. Boston, Harvard University Press, 1971, p 17.

Tomas J. Silber, M.D.

9

PHYSICIAN-ADOLESCENT PATIENT RELATIONSHIP THE ETHICAL DIMENSION

A physician involved in the practice of adolescent medicine needs to be concerned with the ethical dimensions in the physician–patient relationship at that time of life. This chapter analyzes these and addresses the ethical dimension and role models present in their interaction.

THE ADOLESCENT PATIENT-PHYSICIAN RELATIONSHIP

The *adolescent patient* is obviously an abstraction. There are remarkable individual differences among adolescent patients as expressed by age, stage of sexual development, race, social class, health, etc. Nevertheless, all have one thing in common: they are facing their second period of individuation.[1] They have developmental tasks to fulfill. These universal tasks have been described as: . . . "the adolescent has enforced upon him the invariable task of moving from his family of origin to a different (his own) family of procreation; to assume adult procreative function, he must sever close ties with the nuclear family and establish them with blood strangers. Another common denominator is the change from being nurtured to providing

Reprinted by courtesy of Clinical Pediatrics 19(1):50, 1980.

nurture."[2] To this may be added the task of developing and reassessing their own value system.[3]

It is within this context that adolescents become patients, either by their own will or having been brought in by others. Understanding them and their moral dilemmas can at times be quite difficult, particularly if they do not present their problems in an articulate manner.

The *physician* is also an abstraction. The physician may be the patient's pediatrician, gynecologist, family doctor, psychiatrist, emergency room physician, or consultant. Regardless of their background, all physicians share a common obligation to their patients. The nature of this obligation is open to controversy, ranging from "technical" descriptions to "comprehensive medical care." Physicians, however, have an additional and subtle obligation to their adolescent patient, where they transcend the "professional model" and become a model of human being.

THE PHYSICIAN-ADOLESCENT PATIENT RELATIONSHIP

Szasz and Hollender described three basic models of doctor–patient relationships:[4] (1) *Activity–Passivity:* The physician does something to the patient, and the patient is unable to respond. The clinical application of this model can be seen in critical situations, such as during the administration of anesthesia, acute trauma, coma, or delirium. The prototype of this model is the parent–neonatal relationship. (2) *Guidance–Cooperation:* This includes less critical situations. The physician tells the patient what to do, and the patient obeys. The clinical application of this model is well exemplified in acute infectious illness. The prototype of this model is the parent–older child relationship. This model differs from the active–passive relationship, in that both participants are active, contributing to the relationship and what will come from it. But, "the main difference between the two participants pertains to power and to its actual or potential use."[4] Although the patient is assuming some responsibility, the doctor remains clearly dominant. (3) *Mutual Participation:* The physician's role is to help the patient help himself; the patient's role is that of participant in a "partnership" (using expert help). The clinical application of this model can be seen in most chronic illnesses and psychoanalysis. Its prototype is the adult–adult relationship. It is therefore rarely, if ever, appropriate for young children, the mentally defective or those who are very poorly educated. The participants have approximately equal power and need each other. In some ways, the relationship will be satisfactory to both.

Each of these different types of doctor–patient relationships is appropriate for certain circumstances, but how can this typology be applied to the physician–adolescent patient relationship? To answer this, we must assess how the developmental tasks of adolescence are being fulfilled. Depending on "where the patient is," the relationship may fall into one model or another. To have a mutually constructive experience, physicians dealing with adolescent patients will have to undergo in the relationship a process of change which is similar to another quite familiar process: "the need for the parent to behave ever differently toward his growing child."[4]

THE ETHICAL DIMENSION

Having briefly described some basic characteristics of adolescent patients, their physicians, and their kinds of relationships, let us consider the ethical dimension. To illustrate this subject, three ethical problems follow, each involving adolescents and their physicians. They are taken at random from one of the usual busy days in an Adolescent Medicine Program.

Case a. Wanda, age 16, is pregnant. Both she and her boyfriend are in high school and are doing well. She is the only child of a divorced mother. This pregnancy was the result of Wanda's only episode of sexual intercourse. She is anxious, almost desperate. She is considering the possibility of abortion and is troubled by her religious conviction and by fear of pain. She has an intense preoccupation about how her mother is going to feel about her. She asks her doctor for advice.

Case b. John, age 14, has episodes of recurrent abdominal pain. He is hospitalized for evaluation. In the course of this hospitalization, he suffers two episodes of pain. After being examined, John is told that a medicine has been found that is going to help. A placebo is given, and the pain is alleviated immediately. His family is then notified that he responded to placebo therapy. Prior to his discharge, the staff notices a lot of giggling and secret murmurings by relatives standing near his room.

Case c. Rhonda, age 18, has her second episode of pelvic inflammatory disease. She receives antibiotics administered intravenously, but does not improve. She is in pain, hostile, and isolated. She criticizes her doctor and nurse for not curing her "as fast as the first time." Her physician reviews the case and finds that the pharmacy has been sending an incorrect, insufficient dose of medication. Should he let her know what happened?

Ethical theory, understood as an attempt to give a rational account of a morality, may provide a satisfactory approach to the physician facing such problems.[5] Ethical theory does not give a concrete answer to specific problems but serves as a guide to how to look for an answer, how to see what factors are relevant. A theory of morality explains decisions, illuminates conclusions, tests for consistency.

Several approaches have enriched moral philosophy; they differ in the criteria utilized to decide what is good. Some theories focus on what will be the *consequence* of a behavior (consequential ethics). Some see pleasure as the deciding criterion (hedonists); others, looking also at the consequences, embrace "the greatest happiness for the greatest number" (utilitarianism). Another viewpoint has been taken in the so-called "self-development ethics" in which the "right" behavior is the one that promotes self-realization. The formalists, on the other hand, appeal to the concept of deonthologic ethics (from the Greek word for "duty"). They state that the rightness of the act does not flow from the goodness of the consequences of the act, but rather from looking at the *character of the act.*

How does all this apply to the adolescent patient and his physician? It applies, in that morality is put to test every day in our offices and hospitals. Moral problem-solving requires that a logical sequence of reasoning be applied to a situation in which an answer is required and in which there is no immediate source of reliable information. The process may take place either consciously or unconsciously. When we answer a moral problem we obviously don't do a review of ethical theory. Each of us has a morality, a set of principles and values which normally guide our actions. These principles are enmeshed in complicated ways. Although we may not be fully aware or conscious of them, they point toward a logical sequence.

The knowledge of ethical theory may be very useful to practicing physicians, by assisting them, for example, to aid in solving moral problems, sometimes by merely helping the adolescents to articulate their questions. At other times, it may be helpful in seeing if they asked the right question. A doctor can often assist the patient in looking at the conflict among competing alternatives or frameworks.

In brief, it is by our analysis of patient needs, by our skill and persistence in addressing them, by the atmosphere conducive to moral growth that we try to provide in our office or hospital, by the discussion in which we are willing to engage, and by our stance toward their surrounding society that we can and do influence our patients' moral growth.

Even more important than the act of counseling and of value clarification is therefore the doctor's example: the doctor as a role model.

DISCUSSION

Returning to the three examples, we may look at their ethical dimension. In Case a, Wanda is faced by a choice. The unwanted pregnancy highlights a problem that is often present in the doctor–patient relationship: the need to address "ethically charged" material. Some questions arise immediately. What does it mean to be nonjudgmental? What is the adolescent's responsibility? What are the doctors' obligations? It is important to stress that to be nonjudgmental does not mean to relinquish one's own values, nor to be blind or indifferent to the ethical. It doesn't mean to psychologize ethics as a "nothing but" entity. Being "nonjudgmental" means to do one's utmost to be objective. An essential part of objectivity is avoiding the imposition of one's personal value judgments on the patient. In response to Wanda's plea for advice, her physician helped her to continue her inquiry. Her questions included, "Is there something I ought to do?" "How do I feel about it?" "How will I feel ten years from now?" "Which decision will make me less miserable?" "What kind of person will this make me?" Obviously, Wanda learned that there was no easy solution. Wanda entered the realm of moral reasoning. Without knowing it, she retraced the steps of deontologists, consequentialists, and self-realization theorists. Wanda compared her reasoning with her moral intuition and made her decision.

In Cases b and c, it is the doctor who has a choice. He has to face what he thinks is right. The questions that come up relate to his obligation toward the patient, the consequences of the action, and the best interest of the patient. In John's case, the physician had two intentions in prescribing the placebo: diagnostic, to differentiate between "real" and "functional" pain, and therapeutic, to eliminate pain. He did not contemplate the implicit deception and lack of respect of the procedure toward John as a person (deontologic argument). He also overlooked the loss of trust resulting from the deception (consequential argument).

In the case of Rhonda, on the other hand, the physician chose to tell her the truth candidly. He sensed that in order to obtain collaboration from the patient, the relationship had to continue along with the mutual-participation model, which must include sharing the real reason for her lack of improvement.

What constituted the ethical dimension? In these, as well as in so many other situations, a choice had to be made, often in circumstances that were not totally the responsibility of the people involved. A significant decision had to be made. There was impact on others and on one's own life that was important. Decisions were made after exploration of key principles, values, and loyalties, and after questioning what the consequences of alternate decisions were likely to be.

At the end of such process, doctors and patients often agree on shared values such as: respect for truth as a definable moral value and faith in the free play of critical intelligence; respect for the basic worth, equality, and dignity of each individual; recognition of the need for cooperative effort for the common good; and recognition of the right of self-determination of each individual.[6] These general ethical values offer a broad framework that serves as a guideline helping to choose among competing ethical criteria and competing alternative decisions.

REFERENCES

1. Blos P: On Adolescence: A Psychoanalytic Interpretation. New York, Macmillan Co., 1962.
2. Committee on Adolescence, Group for the Advance of Psychiatry: Normal Adolescence. The Scribner Library, 1968.
3. Kohlberg L, Gillian C: The adolescent as a philosopher: Daedalus. Am Acad Arts Sciences, Boston, Massachusetts, Fall 1971.
4. Szasz T, Hollender M: A contribution to the philosophy of medicine. AMA Arch Intern Med 97:585, 1956.
5. Melden AI: Ethical Theories: A Book of Readings with Revisions. Englewood Cliffs, NJ, Prentice-Hall, 1967.
6. Nye I: Values, family and a changing society. J Marriage Family 22:241, 1967.

1. Hunt R, Arras J (eds): Ethical Issues in Modern Medicine. Palo Alto, CA, Mayfield, 1979.
2. Marsh FH: The Deeper Meaning of Confidentiality Within the Physician/Patient Relationship. Ethics Sci Med, 6:131, 1979.
3. Reiser SJ, Dyke AJ, Curran WJ (eds): Ethics in Medicine: Historical Perspectives and Contemporary Concerns. Cambridge, MA, The MIT Press, 1977.
4. Ramsay P: The Patient as Person. New Haven, Yale University Press, 1970.
5. Shannon TA: Bioethics. New York, Paulist Press, 1976.

SECTION FOUR

SPECIAL PROBLEMS

There are a multitude of ethical problems that confront the pediatrician in his daily practice. This section starts with Silber's observations on the morality of the use of placebo therapy. Jean Carlin follows, presenting a series of intriguing concerns relating to the ethics of adoption. Robert Cooke develops the right of the mentally retarded to normalization. He considers in his chapter the theme of sexual freedom under normalization, deinstitutionalization, least restrictive alternatives (LRA), mainstreaming, guardianship, and surveillance. To conclude this section, Silber chose to highlight the application of moral reasoning to the subject of adolescent sexuality. This includes a discussion of the role of the pediatrician as counselor, and the distinction between medical facts and moral rules, as well as between moral dilemmas and pseudoethical dilemmas. It concludes with the controversial subject of the ethical considerations in the medical care of adolescents who seek contraceptive services.

Tomas J. Silber, M.D.

10

PLACEBO THERAPY THE ETHICAL DIMENSION

In requesting a medline search on the subject of placebos in English, German, and Spanish (1976 to 1978), I was surprised by the existence of 1500 articles. When I looked at the number of articles dealing with the ethics of placebo administration, I was surprised again—only 18 of those articles dealt with that issue. There is incongruity between the richness of the pharmacologic, therapeutic, psychiatric, and research literature on this subject in general and the scant attention paid to the moral issues involved. The understanding of the ethical dimension of the diagnostic and therapeutic use of placebos would benefit from more precise examination.

DEFINITIONS

First, what is meant by placebo, impure placebo, and placebo effect? "Placebo" (Latin for "I shall please") is defined in *Webster's New Collegiate Dictionary* (1977) as "a medication prescribed more for the mental relief of the patient then for its actual effect on his disorder." *Dorland's Illustrated Medical Dictionary* describes the placebo as "an inactive substance or preparation given to satisfy the patient's symbolic need for drug therapy, and used in controlled studies to determine the efficacy of medicinal substances." Leslie specifies further: "A placebo is a medicine or preparation which has no inherent pertinent pharmacological activity but which is effective only by virtue of the factor of suggestion attendant upon its administration. The substance may be ingested, injected, inserted, inhaled, or applied."[1] Shapiro gives the broadest definition: "Any therapy (or component of therapy) that is deliberately or knowingly used for its nonspecific, psychologic or psychoprophylactic effect."[2] "Impure placebo," also called "active placebo," differs from the placebo in that it contains a substance with some inherent pharmacologic activity not relevant to the immediate problem to be treated. The "placebo effect" has been defined as "the effect of any therapeutic procedure or component thereof which objectively does not have any specific activity for the condition being treated."[3]

HISTORIC ANTECEDENTS

We lack any historic record of philosophic thought as it relates to placebo administration. There are, though, some glimpses, as in the famous remark by Plato: "A lie is useful only as a medicine to men. The use of such medicines should be confined to physicians" (from *The Republic*). Medicine as a modern science is a recent development, while medicine as an art has a long history. The first cures produced a concept: some substances under some circumstances alleviate suffering. Many of the first physicians perhaps were not aware of the placebo effect, and they attributed cures to the effectiveness of their medications (eg, animal excretions, spermatic fluids of dogs, and herbs). The early medical literature fails to mention placebos as such. Only in the last two centuries, with the advancement of clinical science, has a clear distinction emerged between the active substance that performs through a pharmacologic process and the inert substance that acts through suggestion. These studies led to the discovery of adverse side effects of placebos, placebo addiction, and placebo reactors, among others.[3-5]

COMMENT

When faced with a situation wherein the physician has the choice to use a placebo, a series of questions arises in addition to the medical issue, such as the following: What is included in the obligation toward the patient? What is the best interest of the patient? What are the short- and long-term consequences of the action? What is the influence of the practice on the community? How does it affect professional ethics? These questions may be best understood if they are viewed in the context of an underlying assumption: there is one fundamental principle determining if an action is morally right.

There are two schools of thought in ethics competing for a supreme principle. One looks at the consequence of an act and therefore at the balance, eg, the patient who gets much better with placebo therapy vs the treating nurse who loses confidence in physicians. The other looks at the nature of the act in itself, eg, deceit involved. The former may be described as an utilitarian view, the latter as a deontologic view.

There is also another approach to this problem, and this is the traditional view of many practitioners (Aristotelian): it is the good man who will do the good work. The preponderant thought accordingly goes: The virtuous physician will use placebo virtuously. The main issue is to be—become a good physician. To introduce order into the numerous positions expressed in relationship to the ethical aspects of placebo use, I propose for practical purposes to divide them into two groups: those that build down and those that build up. The first position considers placebo therapy as morally wrong and permissible only in cases of tremendous need when there seems to be no better alternative. The second viewpoint assumes no prohibition against placebo therapy and builds up from this lenient position to safeguard against indiscriminate use of placebos.

Building down is elucidated by Bok, condemning, on deontologic grounds, the use of placebos.[6] She recommends their use only (1) after careful diagnostic workup, when no other agents are known to be effective, (2) without prescribing any active drugs, (3) without lying, and (4) under no circumstances to those who have requested not to receive them. The author's concern is that the physician who is likely to use placebos will eventually abuse them. Cabot states that patients have learned to expect medicine for every symptom and that they have learned this from their physicians.[7] He makes his viewpoint clear: "It is we physicians who are responsible for perpetuating false ideas about disease and its cure . . . with every placebo that we give, we do our part in perpetuating error, a harmful error at that!"

Building up is demonstrated by Leslie, acknowledging that the administration of placebos constitutes a deception; but he draws a fine line between deceit and deception.[1] (The latter is being justified for the welfare of the patient.) He makes an analogy between the use of placebo and the dilemma of truth-telling. His indications for placebo therapy are as follows: weaning patients off narcotics and sedatives; for terminally ill patients, interpolating placebo with active pain relievers to lessen constipation and respiratory depression; as a substitute for a group of drugs a patient might be taking when they cloud the clinical picture; and as a temporary concession to a patient who cannot wait until the end of his diagnostic evaluation. Collard advocates a liberal use of placebo, claiming that its regular use is justified because of its effectiveness (utilitarian viewpoint).[8]

Obviously the ethical dimension of placebo therapy remains controversial. I will use this opportunity to share some thoughts with the reader. My purpose here is to elicit responses and further contributions on the difficult issue of the morality of placebo therapy. The first thought is that at a minimum, whenever placebos are medically contraindicated, this implies an ethical prohibition. Examples are when they are merely a convenience for the physician replacing a needed evaluation, when they are used for diagnostic purposes (the margin of error is extremely high), and when appropriate specific therapy is available. (All of the reasoning that applies to placebo therapy extends to impure placebos with an additional moral problem: the patient is submitted to the dangers and side effects of active agents that were not needed in the first place.) The second thought proposes to look at placebo therapy as an act of communication. This relates to Paracelsus' original view that it is the medical act in its totality that has its effect on the patient. This means that the act of prescribing medication should not be viewed as a separate (and more valuable) segment of the physician–patient relationship. The particular act of prescribing a placebo should be looked at in its totality, including the intention as part of the act. It is conceivable that in some circumstances, and this probably is much more true in the psychiatric field, the act of giving-receiving the placebo implies a special form of communication, a symbolic communication reminiscent of the religious communion. The laying on of hands as well as the giving of something to be incorporated by mouth are indeed powerful ways of communication that say something that words cannot say at one particular moment. In the nature of this phenomenon, I see a justification for placebo therapy.

Last, but not least, when placebo therapy is given, it needs to be part of a careful clinical plan moving actively in the direction of health. Thus, placebo therapy is accepted as moral when it enhances physician-patient communication, and it is accompanied by active efforts to achieve health. Conversely, placebo therapy is viewed as immoral if it diminishes or replaces patient–physician communication and there is no genuine pursuit of health.

REFERENCES

1. Leslie A: Ethics and practice of placebo therapy. Am J Med 16:854–862, 1954.
2. Shapiro AK: Factors contributing to the placebo effect. Am J Psychiatry 18:73–88, 1964.
3. Wolf S, Pinsky RH: Effects of placebo administration in (comparison with mephenesin) and occurrence of toxic reactions. JAMA 155:339–341, 1954.
4. Aznar-Ramos R, Giner-Velázquez J, Lara-Ricalde R, et al: Incidence of side effects with contraceptive placebo. Am J Obstet Gynecol 105:1144–1149, 1969.
5. Vinar O: Dependence on placebo: A case report. Br J Psychiatry 115:1189–1190, 1969.
6. Bok S: The ethics of giving placebos. Sci Am 231:17–23, November 1974.
7. Cabot RC: The use of truth and falsehood in medicine: An experimental study. Am Med 5:344–349, 1903.
8. Collard J: A sociopsychological approach to the placebo effect. Rev Med Liege 32(pt 2):334–339, 1977.

Jean E. Carlin, M.D., Ph.D.

11

ETHICAL PROBLEMS RAISED BY ADOPTION

The ethical issues involved in child care and placement have recently begun to be of concern to physicians and to society in general. Children and women were considered, along with animals, to be possessions, and, consequently, the issue of rights did not arise until relatively recently in history.

In the United States, the privilege of voting was extended to nonwhite groups in 1868 (14th Amendment) and 1870 (15th Amendment) and finally to women in 1920 (19th Amendment). The 1960s saw the very active emergence of civil rights for blacks, which has subsequently been extended to all racial and ethnic minorities and by extension to other oppressed persons such as women and the handicapped. Lagging far behind were a significantly underrepresented group: children. (Laws preventing cruelty to animals and guaranteeing their humane treatment preceded child abuse laws.)

Until children were recognized as persons and not possessions of their parents, the rights of children (even the rights of the unborn to be born or not to be born) were not addressed because these rights were not even defined. (Rights did not "exist," if children were nonpersons.)

The legal precedents involving children's rights have opened a Pandora's box of problems regarding decisions made for and about children. Among these problem areas is the area of adoption.

Adoption, which is in itself a legal procedure, is defined thus: "to *choose* or take as one's own; to accept into a close dependent relationship," and "to choose or accept."[1] This choice seems historically to have been unilateral and not reversible. That is, the adoptive parents choose to accept the child, and they do not have much time (in some states six months) to change their minds before the adoption is finalized. For a variety of reasons the biologic parents, if alive, have made the decision to relinquish the child for adoption.[2]

Infants and children who have been adopted rarely, if ever, have had any voice in the decisions that affect their lives profoundly. (Occasionally, children who are part of the adoptive family are consulted regarding the adoption of a new child, but an infant or young child to be adopted rarely, if ever, has a choice of siblings or parents.) Apparently, this is a result of the infant or young child's inability to make an informed decision and is no different from the lack of rights of an infant who is with its natural family. As the child grows and matures, its rights demand increasing attention. An attempt to predict what children might require or want or have a right to expect includes avoidance of the loss of any part of the biologic family that could possibly and reasonably be avoided (ie, placement with close relatives when appropriate; placement of siblings together as a very high priority; and always avoiding separation of twins and triplets to provide emotional support, with extremely rare exceptions), thus minimizing the total number of changes in the child's life. This decreases the number of adjustments necessary to prevent serious emotional damage. Follow-up studies, discussed later, could provide a basis for including the child's probable wants early in these decisions.

Minimizing the number of changes in a child's life might be different for the newborn who has not known a family, versus the infant or young child who has already known a family. However, for either the newborn or the young child, this priority might be interpreted to imply that adoptive families should match birth families in socioeconomic level, education, race, religion, age, number of siblings, and so forth. There are significant ethical issues that would arise out of such a practice. Is it fair to a child to place him or her in a home of low socioeconomic status just because the birth home was of a low socioeconomic level (which could not afford to keep him or her) when an equally acceptable one of higher socioeconomic level is available? Conversely, should a family of high socioeconomic level receive a baby for adoption in preference to one of lower socioeconomic level simply because the former home could afford more things for the baby? Should the adoptive home be of the same religious (or nonreligious) background as the birth family? Should political convictions or race or ethnicity be major determinants? Should all handicaps in the adoptive parents exclude them from adopting a child? Should age of adoptive parents match birth parents' ages? Must adoptive parents be married, or can single persons adopt a child? Clearly, some of these questions become absurd, since some are part of the reason the birth parent(s) could not keep the child; some are probably irrelevant; some are definitely discriminatory; and so forth. It is my opinion that we need carefully controlled follow-up studies on the effects of these parameters in order to try to be responsive to the needs and rights of adopted children in the future. Some research on cross-racial adoptions has been done by Schecter and Sorosky and by Simon and Altstein.[4,5] Some unique problems occur in cross-racial and cross-cultural adoptions.

What are the rights of birth parents in determining what kind of adoptive home their baby will have? Do birth parents' rights take precedence over adoptive parents' rights and desires or over children's needs and rights as predicted from the above-mentioned follow-up studies? Can they place such restrictive conditions on the adoption that babies and children cannot be placed for adoption if such conditions cannot be met? Can they delay indefinitely in making a decision to give the child up for adoption, thus in my opinion, condemning a child indefinitely to a series of foster homes and denying the child any opportunity to have a stable home and family of its own?[6] Can birth parents change their minds and reclaim their child at a later date after adoption? Do they have the right to contact the child after adoption? And what happens to grandparents' rights to see and know their biologic grandchild?[7] The biologic parents and grandparents do have needs, but the child and the adoptive parents and adoptive grandparents have needs also. Perhaps each case requires some individualized decisions; ultimately the child's needs and rights should take precedence.

Do adopted children have the right to reject the adoption as they become older and realize that they are adopted, if they are dissatisfied with their adoptive families (or are these families analogous to birth families, which children legally may not vote to reject?). If any child has a family that abuses or rejects him or her, that child may need another home, and the social agencies must be able to provide aid. Rejection of the family as part of adolescent rebellion needs careful counseling, however, and not removal. Do adoptive children have the right to inherit from adoptive parents?[8] Is this inheritance by adopted children the same as for the family's own biologic children? In some states, adoptive parents do not inherit from adopted children automatically (to protect the child); yet, adopted children do inherit from adoptive parents.[9] Do adopted children have any claim to inheritance from their birth parents, and do birth parents retain any inheritance rights from their biologic but now adopted child?[10]

Does the adopted child have a right to search for and contact his or her biologic parents?[11,12] If so, at what age is this a "right," and what conditions apply? The usual age is after 18 years, and that is probably an acceptable decision for all concerned. What rights do the biologic parents have regarding whether or not they are to be contacted? Must the biologic parents live in fear that some day, against their wishes, they will be found and contacted? The programs that aid in these searches do offer the right not to be contacted, and I think this is good. Must adoptive parents cooperate with their child's search for its "other" or "real" parents? Must the adoptive parents tell the adopted child what they know about the biologic parents if the child and they (the adoptive parents) might be badly hurt by this?[13]

In fact, should children always be told that they are adopted? What are the pros and cons of this? Is it a child's right to know this information? (And if it is, what about the rights of test tube babies, artificial insemination babies, and children of surrogate mothers; and what about the rights of the adults in these situations?) Adopted children almost always sense and find out about their adoption in some way. I think it is better, usually, if the adoptive parents tell them. Some facts may be withheld if they would damage the child; however, genetic information is needed by the child for future decisions.

In addition, do adoptive parents have the right to "return" or void an adoption if the child turns out to have physical or mental handicaps or emotional problems? Can adoptive (or biologic) parents reject their offspring if it is not convenient to keep them anymore?

The issues of giving or withholding proxy consent for medical procedures or schooling for minor children have demanded public attention. Do adoptive parents and biologic parents *own* their minor children's lives? Do adoptive and biologic children and their earnings or gifts belong to the parents regardless of the children's desires? If so, which parents? In some states, children's earnings and belongings (ie, a car purchased by a minor child 16 or 17 years old with money earned by that child) can be taken and used or sold by the parents even against the minor child's wishes.[14] Are these indeed within the scope of adoptive (or biologic) parents' rights?

Who protects the child's rights? Who protects the adoptive parents' rights? Who protects the biologic parents' rights? Who protects the rights of biologic or adoptive siblings? Who mediates when these various rights are in conflict?

What are the problems when adoptions involve homes with very different religious convictions or homes of different and obvious racial or ethnic differences? What problems occur in interracial and/or international adoptions?

Perhaps it is not entirely accidental that the numerous questions raised in this chapter have only recently been given attention. This whole area has represented an unconscious threat to society and has been actively repressed until great human suffering and recent litigation focused our attention on this neglected area.

REFERENCES

1. Corpus Juris Secundum #140: Adoption of Persons.
2. Corpus Juris Secundum #57: Adoption of Persons.
3. Sokoloff B: Current issues in adoption: An overview. Proc Int Conf Adoles, Edinburgh, Scotland, 1976, pp 44–51.
4. Schecter M, Sorosky A: Cross-Racial Adoption. South Carolina, South Carolina Psychiatric Society.
5. Simon R, Altstein H: Transracial Adoption. New York, John Wiley & Sons, Inc., 1977.
6. Sokoloff B: Adoption and foster care—the pediatrician's role. Pediatrics in Review, 57–61, 1979.

7. Kornhaber A: Grandparents-Children's Rights. Haslett, MI.
8. Corpus Juris Secundum #149.
9. Corpus Juris Secundum #146: Inheritance from Natural Parents.
10. Corpus Juris Secundum #151: Inheritance from Adopted Child.
11. Sokoloff B: Should the adoptive adolescent have access to his birth records and to his birth parents? Clin Ped 16:975–977, 1977.
12. Sokoloff B: Adoptive families needs for counseling. Clin Ped 18:184–190, 1979.
13. Sorosky AD, Baran A, Pannor R: The reunion of adoptees and birth relatives. J Youth Adoles 3(3):195–206, 1974.
14. Corpus Juris Secundum #102.

Robert E. Cooke, M.D.

12

ETHICS ON BEHALF OF THE MENTALLY RETARDED

All the mentally retarded need is a bench to sit on and a lollypop to suck.

—Superintendent, State Training School, 1937

All the mentally retarded need is a three-bedroom house in the suburbs, house parents, four sibs, and possibly a dog or cat.

—Description of normalization, 1981

The changes over the last 40 years in the ideal environment for the retarded seem monumental, even if the above statements are only approximations to reality. Deinstitutionalization is accelerating—not rapidly, but grudgingly, as advocacy groups work and legal efforts continue to be made on behalf of the retarded. Yet it is progressing, and the principle underlying all such efforts to deinstitutionalize the retarded is that of normalization.

Despite change, however, it is still not clear that society in general, or even professionals in the field, know what the goal of normalization is or why it is being carried out. Are the purposes clear? Is the answer simply that the trappings of daily living should be different from years ago, as the quotations above illustrate?

It is the purpose of this chapter to analyze the ethical issues underlying normalization, to examine what the least-restrictive alternative means ethically, to determine what problems exist for guardianship, and to indicate what the programmatic consequences are of the differing ethical perceptions.

Reprinted by courtesy of Pediatric Annals 10:24, 1981.

Such a discussion is obviously not as spectacular as other ethical issues related to mental retardation, such as the right to survive or die, the right to education, the right to marry, or the ethics of sterilizing the mentally retarded person, and the ethics of human experimentation, or consent, or behavior modification.

Normalization is the major theme of public policy, however. It is the dominant note in the rash of consent decrees emanating from the courts. It is the basis of the nationwide deinstitutionalization effort—the primary reason for the development of community care. It underlies the concept of the least-restrictive alternative and of mainstreaming. Hence, it is essential for the care of the retarded that the ethical basis of normalization be clearly understood by all professionals in the field, because the concept is so pervasive.

It is doubly important for pediatricians to understand this since pediatricians, increasingly, are expected to be experts in mental retardation even though it is still but a small facet of the usual pediatric practice. More important, the ethical issues relating to normalization closely resemble those related to growing up, to the process of becoming an independent, autonomous, normal adult.

The issues of normalization are morally similar to those of child-rearing, particularly during adolescence. "Adultification" and normalization have many ethical issues in common. Certainly the field of child development has contributed much to the care of the retarded and, to an extent, the converse is true.

The earliest proponents of normalization came from the Scandinavian countries and emphasized the importance of the physical environment in the process of normalization. Wolf Wolfensberger, who popularized the concept in the United States, stressed assisting the retarded to be as normal as possible.[2] From these origins normalization has come to be perceived from two distinct ethical perspectives. The differences between the two seem morally significant and need analysis.

NORMALIZATION I

Normalization may be considered as the process by which the retarded are helped to become as normal-appearing, -behaving, -living, as possible so that they become indistinguishable from the rest of society. The environment becomes the critical factor. Hence, every effort is made to assure that the living environment resembles that of most American families. Large groups of retarded persons are not allowed in any community residential complex. Isolation is also forbidden. Houses are required to be indistinguishable from others in the neighborhood. No appearance of an institutional setting is allowed. The interiors are expected to be decorated just as any other private residence. The decor of rooms is adult in character. Child-appropriate possessions are discouraged. Training for useful employment, for everyday living is considered essential. The common virtues of reliability, industry, punctuality, neatness, pleasantness, compliance, temperance, and moderation are inculcated.

This "model of virtue" is cultivated and trained, not for its own sake, but with the belief that the retarded can best be integrated into and accepted by society if they are as perfect as we would all wish to be—if they produce the fewest waves. The more the behavior of the retarded is accepted, it is believed, the better and the more frequent the opportunities they will have.

From such a perspective, the adult retarded person is expected to adhere to the work ethic, to eschew sex, usual or unusual, and to avoid drinking alcoholic beverages, at least in public. The environment is carefully controlled to prevent undue risk of physical harm and psychologic harm from temptation and to minimize aberrant behavior. The patient, or client, is expected to conform to rules which are imposed by professionals, parents, or other lay people and which are believed to be in his or her best interest.

Behavior is expected to be age appropriate. Childlike activities and wishes are discouraged. Choosing is not forbidden, but nonconforming choices are not acted upon so that the retarded is spared hardships. If a client does not wish to bathe every day, or he does not like his work experience, he is labeled as uncooperative and the modifiers of behavior are called in. If the retarded client exhibits aggressive behavior, uses foul language or socializes excessively or not at all, he is considered a problem. The supervisory system is not considered too rigid or demanding; only the client is maladapted, and he may be banished from his vocational training if he does not comply. Compliance soon becomes the primary virtue just as in the institution. Options are provided only when it is judged by some authority that a correct decision will be made.

Guardianship is encouraged so that adequate protection is provided in order that the retarded person's resources will not be wasted. Regardless of the loss of friends or familiar environment, the retarded is required, frequently by court action, to leave the institution and live with three or four strangers in a community residence, even though the chances of finding compatible acquaintances are small. Because a building large enough to house 10 to 20 residents is not a typical family setting, it is not acceptable, even though friendships may be easier to establish.[3] It is little appreciated that three or four normal persons may live together in a community because they choose to do so, because they enjoy the companionship of their chosen friends, not because they are placed there.

Throughout such an approach to normalization is the sincere desire to maximize good and minimize harm. This perspective sees the greatest good for the retarded, for his family, and for society, coming from his being made as normal as possible. The emphasis is on protection and direction, less, of course, for the less severely handicapped but protection, nevertheless. Emphasis is placed on the least-restrictive alternative rather than on maximum freedom compatible with safety. Efforts are made to ease limits, not to expand opportunities. The intent is to assure that the consequences are good and in the best interest of the retarded.

The other concept of normalization is based less on consequential reasoning and more on respect for the retarded as persons. Persons are thought of as independent, autonomous, self-controlling, decision-making individuals. Respect for persons demands respect for the decision-making capacities of people. Choosing becomes an essential feature of being a person.

Normalization from this perspective means the provision of opportunities for choosing, for independent decision-making, for autonomy—full or limited. The emphasis is placed on providing opportunities to choose, regardless of whether or not the decisions are the same as those that normal persons would make.

Normalization in this context need not require a normal environment, although that might be highly effective.[4,5] It definitely requires a series of training efforts, not to make the retarded person act like everyone else, but to provide understandable options, to provide information that allows a reasonable choice, to provide practice and encouragement in making choices. The process of preparation of a retarded person for deinstitutionalization, or the preparation of a child in the home for community placement, becomes one of improving communication skills of all concerned (not just of the retarded) so that options are understood and choices are expressed and properly appreciated. Just as important is the full understanding by the retarded person of the consequences of his choices. It is not enough to permit only choices that are acceptable to the caretakers, since normalization in this context means choosing as normal people may, and normal people are allowed a wide variety of choices. The retarded, to profit from his mistakes, must to an extent live with the consequences of his choices.

It is not difficult to perceive the complications that can and do arise with such an interpretation of the normalization principle. For example, if a retarded adult does not like the attitudes of the staff of the workshop, what can he do? The normal worker has a number of options available, including that of looking for other employment. If the retarded person's dissatisfaction is demonstrated by acting-out behavior, he is labelled as uncooperative. Efforts are redoubled to make the client more compliant, or he may be dropped from the workshop (with no other facilities for training or employment available). Alternatively, psychiatric intervention is ordered, with or without psychotropic agents, or intense behavior modification efforts may be prescribed.

If the retarded person uses his limited earnings for something as frivolous as an alcoholic beverage, he may be considered irresponsible and such a "privilege" as managing his own finances will be curtailed. Frequently, taverns and bars are considered off limits for retarded clients because of the possibility of their exposure to undesirable influences. Although caretaking staffs are not so limited, drunkenness in retarded clients evokes much justifiable concern.

The problems become more and more complex with greater degrees of retardation. Communication is more difficult, choices are hard for the retarded person to explain and even more difficult for the staff or parents to comprehend. Risks or harm from unreasonable choices are considerable, and serious harm may occur if adequate restrictions and limits are not imposed. Who imposes such limits? Who, and by what criteria the constraints are monitored become important questions.

Self-improvement is frequently assumed to be a basic principle by which most of us operate. Efforts to improve one's self are considered highly virtuous. In the absence of such efforts, persons are thought of as lazy, poorly motivated, without ambition, even disturbed or disordered. Yet if a normal person chooses to drop out of training or school (after an imposed minimum), that is his misfortune. Relatively little is done to correct the situation.

By contrast, if the retarded person drops out of training, his developmental progress may cease and his caretakers frequently will force continuation through various measures despite his objections, on behalf of his best interest. It is not surprising then, that behavioral difficulties or psychiatric illnesses arise in a high percentage of retarded persons. Yet, their rewards for self-improvement are meager. Doing well in the workshop brings few meaningful advantages over doing poorly. If childish activities are more enjoyable, how should the caretakers respond? How soon should the modifiers of behavior be called in to effect necessary changes? If an adult client prefers to keep her dolls and her childhood play things in a "normalized" room in her "normalized" community residence, what should be done? Her caretakers might be cited as inadequate by the monitors of her consent decree from the court that has ordered her deinstitutionalization based on the normalization principle. It is a difficult problem to judge how fully a child's mind in an adult's body should be respected.

If an adult client prefers to remain in his own home rather than live independently in a community residence with his peers, how vigorously should one push for a more normal (age-appropriate) environment? Parents, as well as institutional caretakers, may severely limit the opportunities for choice in the care of their retarded children because they wish to protect their child from harm and unhappiness resulting from the uncertainties of life.

The dilemma that exists may be summarized in a few words: If normalization is interpreted as making the retarded appear normal, serious infringement of personal autonomy is necessary. If normalization is interpreted as encouraging choosing as normal persons can, then developmental progress may be slowed and other undesirable consequences may result as well.

GUIDELINES FOR CARING FOR THE MENTALLY RETARDED

It would be unfortunate if we made no effort to resolve such a difficult situation. It should be helpful to caretakers and to their advisors, such as pediatricians, to provide some approximate guidelines for the care of the mentally retarded in the community.

1. The efforts of all caretakers should resemble those of parents of normal adolescents—namely, to encourage the maximum number of decisions compatible with personal safety. In preparation for such opportunities, decision-making experiences must be provided that can be safely implemented regardless of the quality of the decision. Such choices must be related to their consequences in order to develop responsible decision-making, namely, ascertaining consequences before actions and living with the consequences. Learning from experience is essential for the retarded as well as for the normal person. With the more severely retarded, communication skills should be strengthened. Caretakers, likewise, need to improve their sensitivity to the nonverbal messages transmitted by retarded persons.

2. Programs that provide care should be oriented toward conformity. Such differences should still be compatible with the adequate functioning of the total organization or the family. Responsibility toward others is a trait to be encouraged, obviously, as a part of the development of individual autonomy.

3. Because of the limited adaptive capacity of the retarded person (by definition), adaptation *to* the client by the staff member or family member is necessary rather than expecting major changes to occur in him or her. Nevertheless, future improvement may require change by the retarded person as well. Ideal staff behavior, not unlike ideal parental behavior, becomes one of listening rather than telling, of understanding rather than ordering. The consequences of such behavior will not be anarchy, but rather mutual development as the retarded person progresses gradually toward the attainment of autonomy.

SEXUAL FREEDOM UNDER NORMALIZATION

Environmental normalization provides living arrangements in which males and females may live in close proximity in small community residences. Normalization from the perspective of choosing encourages choosing as normal persons can.

Living together or choosing to be with the opposite sex, however, poses difficult problems. Nowhere does there seem to be more confusion than in relation to sexual freedom of the retarded. The options of intercourse, prostitution, marriage, or homosexual activity are discouraged even though the employment of homosexuals as staff cannot and should not be prohibited legally.

Frequently, the retarded are thought to be sexually overactive, to be a threat to normal people in the community, to be without self-control. Indeed, the opposite seems to be the case. Sterility is relatively common in the retarded population—Down's syndrome is a particular example. Although masturbation may persist actively into adult life since no other sexual outlet is provided, public masturbation is unusual and fairly easily controlled with simple behavioral measures.

Under either concept of normalization, the handling of decisions regarding sexual activities poses problems, particularly in adolescence. Caretakers, professional or parental, are sincerely concerned for the well-being of their client or their adolescent child, particularly if the retarded person is a female. It is usually the neighbors who are concerned if the retarded person is a male. Requests for sterilization to protect the young woman or the community (in the case of the male retarded) still occur with some frequency. The availability of reversible contraceptive measures has probably somewhat reduced the demand for surgical sterilization. An alternative is sterilization by isolation—that is, reducing all heterosexual social contacts to zero.

Such limitation of movement violates the normalization principle regardless of how it is interpreted ethically; proponents of normalization can advocate sterilization as the least-restrictive alternative even though the retarded person may not fully comprehend the consequences. It is important to realize that other alternatives exist that do not have irreversible consequences. First and foremost, education and training in sexual responsibility is possible and feasible even with moderately retarded clients.

The retarded person may be more sexually responsible than a normal individual of the same age.[6] If sexual exposure is probable and desired by the client, then contraceptives or an intrauterine device can provide protection just as with persons with normal intelligence. David Allen quotes an eminent Catholic gynecologist and late director of the Kennedy Institute in Bioethics, Andre Hellegers, in stating that "there is nothing in Catholic teaching that would preclude the use of contraception in the mentally retarded."[7] The request for such use should come from the person, not from the caretakers. Compliance in the taking of medications does not depend upon superior intelligence. The threat of rape in the minds of caretakers does not warrant the imposition of contraceptives on retarded persons any more than it does in the case of normal adolescents. Sexual abuse is not tolerable, with or without risk of pregnancy, and protection against pregnancy is not a license for neglect in supervision.

Although families may fear sexual encounters for the severely retarded person who has little understanding, such persons seem to need human intimacy, not sexual relations. The self-stimulation of masturbation may diminish markedly as loving care and close physical, not sexual, contact replace the isolation of institutional life.

For the less severely retarded, there is a need for mental-age-appropriate sex education, including use of birth control techniques and parenting information. Unfortunately, relatively little such information is available in appropriate form.

One of the ultimate choices that all normal persons consider is that of marriage. If the principle of normalization is taken seriously, then the marriage of retarded persons should be far more common than is observed at the present time. Whether normalization is regarded as looking and living as normal adults do or choosing as normal people do, marriage is likely to be a relatively common occurrence. Clearly there is much justifiable reluctance to encourage such relationships when there is still substantial dependency. If care and upbringing of children were not a problem, marriage (formally recognized and dignified if not necessarily sanctified cohabitation) would represent an excellent solution for friendship and mutual support of retarded persons even for those moderately severely retarded who wish to lead "normal" heterosexual lives.

The problem of defective offspring as well as the costs of care of normal children who might be produced present problems of utility that are difficult to ignore even though respect for persons—the basis of one view of normalization—would favor the opportunity for choice. It is likely that society has been more restrictive and less respectful of the competence of retarded people to serve as parents than is justified.

Situations do exist, however, when parenting would almost certainly be poor or when a defective infant might certainly be conceived. Under those circumstances sterilization in anticipation of marriage might be presented as an option. How full understanding of the consequences can be assessed or how parents or caretakers should proceed if marriage is decided upon but sterilization is not, is indeed difficult, but efforts should be made to try to effect the fairest solution in concert with the retarded persons.

It is worth remembering that no test of competency as a parent is required of a normal person before he can obtain a marriage license or procreate. Nor is any test to prove freedom from genetic disease required. The number of inadequate parents who have normal intelligence far exceeds the number of inadequate parents who are retarded.

DEINSTITUTIONALIZATION

As indicated previously, the principle of normalization guides most consent decrees following class action suits and most social efforts to close traditional state institutions and replace them with small community residences, apartments, modified group homes, or Medicaid intermediate-care facilities for the mentally retarded. What should be done, however, if the client does not wish to leave friends (caretakers or other clients) or leave the security of the institution for the risks of greater social contact? How vigorously should one try to educate the institutional resident as to the perceived advantages of a normal environment?

Frequently parents of long-term institutionalized retarded persons (particularly the severely and profoundly retarded) object to such transfers. The parents have developed confidence in the caretakers and they see clear-cut authority and responsibility in the superintendent of the institution. They are wary of change to a community system in which provider agencies are dependent upon contracts which may or may not be renewed and where responsibility and authority are diffused and staff turnover is common.

Frequently, community medical and dental services for the handicapped are nonexistent. Not infrequently, parents can see no benefit for their older retarded child in being uprooted and moved to a strange environment, even though the new environment is more homelike. One need not evoke feelings of guilt or fears of being burdened with care in order to appreciate the sincere concern of such parents. Family counseling that properly presents the potential benefits and the possible risks is necessary, and informed consent should be obtained and respected.

LEAST-RESTRICTIVE ALTERNATIVE (LRA)

The concept of the least-restrictive alternative embodies the same dilemmas. This is a doctrine that attempts to provide fewer limits and has led to significant good, but problems still remain, as Marsha Seltzer has pointed out.[7] "There may be a conflict between the goal of producing the greatest degree of behavioral gain (or independent behavior) in an individual and allowing him or her the greatest amount of personal liberty," she notes. "Sometimes, we must limit the first to achieve the second." Such a notion certainly resembles the problems found in normal parenting.

Parents at times may disagree with authorities, particularly in school settings, as to the most appropriate placement for their retarded child. School systems, undoubtedly for fiscal reasons, are progressively reducing their commitment to purchase specialized care for groups of retarded persons or for retarded individuals. The legal argument that is used to justify such action is that court decisions using the normalization principle have ordered that the least-restrictive alternative in education as well as housing be used. It is not clear how a special class in a special school is more restrictive of the liberties of retarded children than their participation in a special class in a regular school or even in a regular class in a regular school. If the development of the child is accelerated by placement in a specialized program then that child's opportunities for choice are expanded and his chances of living a more normal life are increased. Unfortunately, there is little evidence from various educational experiments that justifies either choice on grounds of improved developmental progress.

The concept of the least-restrictive alternative was originally intended to apply to residential placement. In that regard there is accumulating evidence that there is material benefit to retarded persons when they are placed in settings other than large state institutions. However, there is little conclusive evidence that one type of facility or particular grouping of clients is more satisfactory than another, because so many variables are involved. It is assumed that the greater the opportunities for socialization, the greater the degree of social progress. The observation of retarded persons in community residences certainly contributes anecdotal evidence to support this belief.

MAINSTREAMING

The application of the normalization principle to schooling has led to the placement of retarded students in regular classes part or full time in regular schools, under the term *mainstreaming*. Just as with the appplication of the concept of the least-restrictive alternative, there is little critical evidence to support or negate mainstreaming. The argument can be made that the retarded student can benefit from exposure to the behavior of normal students as well as to elevated expectations of teachers. In addition, broad social good is postulated to result from exposing normal children to their retarded colleagues. These approaches have an obvious resemblance to those of civil rights and desegregation. How much effect on the retarded and on this normal population results from these interactions is not known. How much the educational progress of both groups is slowed or accelerated remains to be determined. If educational demands are excessive, however, repeated failure in school performance can only lead to reduced self-esteem and behavioral problems. The economic benefits of mainstreaming are real to the financially hard-pressed school system, but such benefits should not accrue to the detriment of handicapped persons.

Normalization, from this standpoint, means respecting individual differences rather than sameness. In an otherwise intelligent statement about discrimination versus prejudice, Robert Miller makes one surprising error.[8] He states that the purpose of mainstreaming in education is to pretend that differences in children do not matter. The idea behind mainstreaming is exactly the opposite—to recognize differences and to help different children learn and live together. Furthermore, if education is to prepare one for life, mainstreaming appears to be an excellent model for encouraging positive discrimination and reducing prejudice.

GUARDIANSHIP AND SURVEILLANCE

The normalization principle suggests that as much civil liberty as possible be provided for each retarded person. As a consequence, guardianship should be as limited as possible. Until the age of majority, the parents legally function in such capacity. But when legal adulthood is achieved, many retarded in the community are without the protection of guardianship. In state institutions the superintendent has traditionally functioned as guardian. In the community, no such single individual exists. Who can consent for surgery, for example, for the severely retarded in a community residence? Who is the conservator of his property and monies? The need for guardianship—limited to such decisions, not to the day-to-day living of adult clients—is clear. Conservator appointment, rather than guardianship, is all that is needed for the less severely retarded persons who can choose their own lifestyles more readily.

The monitoring and surveillance of the application of the normalization principle has become an industry in itself. At the present time there are Individual Educational Plans (IEPs) under Public Law 94-142, the Education for All Handicapped Children Act; Individual Habilitation Plans (IHPs) under the Developmental Disabilities legislation; Individual Service Plans (ISPs) under various statewide consent decrees, as well as a number of other monitoring systems including Independent Professional Review (IPR) and other alphabetical arrangements.

All such plans are directed at ensuring that parents, students and clients participate in the decision-making process and that provider organizations individualize their approaches. From my own observations, the system in the final analysis depends more upon the integrity, interest, and quality of training of those dealing most intimately with clients than upon the degree of detail in the monitoring instruments. Forms cannot substitute for humanity, sensitivity, experience, and dedication, or for the ethical orientation of the staffs dealing with the clients on a daily basis.

REFERENCES

1. Allen DF, Victoria S: Ethical Issues in Mental Retardation. Nashville, Abington Press, 1979.
2. Wolfensberger W: A new approach to decision-making in human management services. *In* Kugel RB, Wolfensberger W (eds): Changing Patterns in Residential Services for the Mentally Retarded. Washington DC, President's Committee on Mental Retardation, 1969, pp 367–381.
3. Landesman-Dwyer S, Sackett GP, Kleinman JS: Relationship of size to resident and staff behavior in small community residences. Am J Ment Defic 85:8–17, 1980.
4. Romer D, Berkson G: Social ecology of supervised communal facilities for mentally disabled adults. IV. Prediction of social choice. Am J Ment Defic 85:243–252, 1980.
5. Hull, JI, Thompson JC: Predicting adaptive functioning of mentally retarded persons in community settings. Am J Ment Defic 85:253–261, 1980.
6. Tarjan G: Sex: A tri-polar conflict in mental retardation. *In* Exman RK, Meyer CE, Tarjan G (eds): Sociobehavioral Studies in Mental Retardation. Monogr Am Assoc Ment Defic 1:175–183, 1979.
7. Seltzer M: Least restriction: Abstraction, guideline, imperative or paradox. Links 10:2–3, 1980.
8. Shell S: Time. Letter to the editor.

Tomas J. Silber, M.D.

13

ADOLESCENT SEXUALITY: AN ETHICAL ISSUE FOR THE PEDIATRICIAN

MEDICAL FACTS AND MORAL RULES

Adolescent sexuality is not a simple, approachable subject like chickenpox or a sprained ankle, and each pediatrician responds to this phenomenon differently. To start, we are usually unprepared to deal with a child's emerging sexuality. Sometimes this is due to the fact that in many patients changes are gradual and subtle; in others, there is no "chief complaint." The main reason for our reluctance to deal with adolescent sexuality, however, is confusion. Part of this confusion is due to our failure to understand the range of normality in adolescent sexual behavior. It is compounded by the lack of adequate terminology. Many of the words we use carry overtones of judgment or criticism: contrast, for example, the terms "serial monogamy" and "promiscuity"; both of which have been applied to the same adolescent sexual conduct.

Yet our difficulties may not be attributed solely to a poor choice of vocabulary or a lack of understanding. The very nature of our response to sexuality is at the heart of the matter. Of all ethical concerns, those related to sexual issues are the ones that most lend themselves to the highest degree of passion and controversy. On this subject, otherwise calm and rational thinkers often operate at intense irrational levels. This is not surprising if

Reprinted by courtesy of Pediatric Annals 11:728, 1982.

one considers that sexuality has both strong subjective connotations and far-reaching effects on social organization. Throughout history, adolescent sexual behavior has been controlled by rules, often in the form of ethical or religious codes. As pediatricians we are as much influenced as anyone else by moral assumptions current in our society. Therefore, in considering this subject, we have to be alert to the possibility that our professional standing may often lead us to express our personal moral convictions in the terminology of medical science. Confusion between medical facts and moral rules, which was rampant among professionals at the beginning of this century, still occurs in more subtle forms. For instance, a current textbook of psychosexual disorders lists oral sex and masturbation under sexual perversions.[1] Although it is the conservative ideologists who usually invest their moral ideals with medical authority, this same predisposition may also be found among modern radical thinkers.[2] The pediatrician who wishes to be of greatest assistance to the adolescent patient must avoid this position.

THE ADOLESCENT AS A DEVELOPER OF VALUES

Thinking rationally about adolescent sexuality is further complicated by the momentous changes in attitudes toward sexuality that have taken place in America.[3] Pluralism has enhanced the adolescent's reluctance to accept an absolute moral code. Many teenagers now prefer gradually to work out their own rules of conduct. In order to understand how this happens, we must be aware of certain developmental characteristics of the adolescent. In adolescence, there is an intensified emotionality that differs qualitatively from that of the child. This happens because the adolescent's emotions are often experienced as a result of states of the self rather than as a direct correlate to external events. Associated with a heightening of subjective feelings comes the discovery of conflicts among feelings. It is also at this time that the capacity for normal operational reasoning emerges.[4] This is characterized by the transition from thoughts about reality to thoughts about possibility. For the first time in their lives, adolescents become capable of reflective thinking and may synthesize ideas. It is this newly acquired skill that is responsible for the frequent questioning of transmitted values.

To understand an adolescent's ethical thinking, however, we need to be aware not only of the stages of cognition and emotional development but also of the particular stages in moral thought. Cognitive maturity is a necessary but not a sufficient condition for mature moral judgment. This has been studied by Kohlberg, who stratified the adolescent's moral development into several stages.[5] For the sake of conceptual clarity they may be divided into three major categories: preconventional, conventional and post-conventional.

Adolescents in the *preconventional* stage are frequently deprived, developmentally immature, or even moderately retarded. These adolescents are often "well-behaved" and are responsive to our culture's labels of "good" and "bad." They interpret "good" or "bad" in terms of physical consequences (reward-punishment) or in terms of the physical power of those that initiate the rules. For example, a patient in this stage recently told me: "My pregnancy is a bad thing. My father told me that if I become pregnant he will kick me out of the house."

The *conventional* stage is most common in early adolescence. In this stage, maintaining the expectations and rules of the family, group, or nation is perceived as valuable in its own right. The adolescent's concern is not only to conform but also to maintain and justify a social order. An example from another patient: "I have decided against an abortion. I am a Catholic and that would go against the teaching of my church."

The *postconventional* level is sometimes noticed around mid-adolescence but it usually appears (if it does at all) in late adolescence. It is characterized by a strong impulse toward autonomous moral principles which carry their weight apart from the authority of the group. As an illustration I quote yet another patient: "I have decided to have an abortion because I am not ready yet to be a mother. I think it is my duty to be well myself before I can take care of a baby."

From the above, it may be understood that the types of moral development are called "stages" because they represent a developmental sequence. An understanding of the adolescent's stages of development and maturation may facilitate the delivery of care.

THE PEDIATRICIAN AS COUNSELOR

The issue of adolescent sexuality highlights a situation that is often present in the doctor/patient relationship: the need to address "ethically-charged" materials.[6] This need evokes some questions: What does it mean to be "non-judgmental"? What is the adolescent's responsibility? What are the doctor's obligations? What is the role of advice? The American Academy of Pediatrics has tackled these issues and has provided useful guidelines for the practitioner that legitimize counseling as part of the pediatrician's task.[7]

For the purpose of this discussion, counseling may be defined as the process in which an individual is helped by talking with a more experienced person. Implicit in this relationship is a manifestation of trust: trust that the pediatrician will put all of his or her skills in the service of the patient's best interest. But what do we mean by the adolescent patient's best interest? Who decides what this is? The principle of autonomy suggests that under certain circumstances the only one entitled to make this judgment is the adolescent.[8] A logical sequela to such a viewpoint would be that the individual adolescent is the only one able to judge what steps may lead to his or her well-being. As pediatricians we do not always believe that our adolescent patients are the best judges of what will lead to their happiness. Indeed, a recurring theme in medical ethics discussions about "paternalism" is the need to clarify what a patient is requesting and what he or she "really needs." We do know that sometimes, because of emotional distress, ignorance, or confusion, adolescents are in no state to judge their own interests. We hope that our adolescent patients may come to recognize this and trust us to act in the interest of the self that they would be if they were mature. Yet it is in these cases where it is hardest for pediatricians to keep their own values from impinging on a medical decision. The detachment required to distinguish "what is right for him/her" from "what would be right for me" is hard to achieve.

Counseling that concerns ethical questions requires the pediatrician to be nonjudgmental. Being nonjudgmental does not mean relinquishing one's own values, or being blind or indifferent to ethical questions. Being nonjudgmental means to do one's utmost to be objective. An essential part of objectivity is, once more, not to impose personal value judgments on a patient. The reason for taking this position is both ethical and practical. "Imposing values" would violate the patient's autonomy, lead to a power struggle and deprive adolescents of an opportunity to work and exercise their own moral codes. Adolescents should be encouraged to weigh decisions, to investigate alternatives and to choose their own way. By applying this Socratic method, a clinician may induce reflection, and reflection may promote a higher level of moral functioning.

The higher level of functioning will not necessarily produce a "right" answer. It is always possible to do the right thing for the wrong reason. However, for many adolescents, it has been helpful to do moral reasoning, to compare it with their moral intuition, and then to proceed.

MORAL DILEMMAS AND PSEUDOETHICAL DILEMMAS

The pediatrician involved in counseling may categorize the issues in two ways, pseudoethical dilemmas and true ethical dilemmas or conflicts of principles.[9] Pseudoethical dilemmas are situations brought to the pediatrician's attention because the patient and/or family find them difficult to resolve and there is *uncertainty over facts*. They are not true ethical problems because they do not contain conflict over principles. An example might illustrate the nature of a pseudodilemma. An older homosexual adolescent asked, "Is homosexuality an illness? Should I suppress my sexual feelings?" The scientific data on homosexual behavior are scant, incomplete, and controversial. If the pediatrician is successful in being objective and nonjudgmental, this case of counseling would consist of assisting the patient in arriving at his own choice within the framework of his own views. This is not to say that the dilemma might not be painful for an adolescent to resolve, nor would counseling the adolescent be an easy task for the pediatrician. The main burden may come from the fact that data are inadequate.

If, on the other hand, a pediatrician has a moral conviction through which he/she condemns homosexuality on principle, the same situation turns into an ethical dilemma. This is so because the potential exists that the patient might be helped by achieving something that is contrary to the pediatrician's own moral code.

At present the most common situation in which a moral dilemma occurs is presented by adolescent patients requesting contraception from a pediatrician who believes that premarital sex is morally wrong. What can a doctor do under such circumstances? His or her first obligation, once more, is to make a clear distinction between personal moral beliefs and facts. The physician must not present beliefs in the guise of scientific doctrine. This includes the need to insure that the moral conviction not induce selective attention to the available scientic evidence (for instance, grossly exaggerating the risks of oral contraceptives). Thus, the pediatrician counseling the sexually active adolescent may think that premarital sex is wrong and yet also be able to acknowledge that a wide spectrum of contraceptive agents are medically indicated for adolescents engaging in sexual intercourse. It is also perfectly legitimate for those pediatricians to be open about the nature of their conflict and, if need be, offer the patient an opportunity of being referred to another physician.

THE PEDIATRICIAN AS SOCIETAL AGENT

Many ethical dilemmas lead ultimately to one question: What kind of society do we want to be? It is therefore impossible to consider the issue of adolescent sexuality out of the context of contemporary society. Oppenheimer emphasizes this point: "In debate, the choice easily becomes polarized between the vision of a sexually free and happy society into which only wanted children are born (or the opposing view, an anarchic society where sex is divorced from love and selfish hedonism prevails), and the vision of a tranquil and decent society in which family life is revered and innocence cherished (or the opposing view, a jealous, repressed society in which human error carries heavy penalties for those least to blame)."[10] This type of concern is of a particular nature. It does not relate exactly to known facts or to value judgments. It deals with the process of changes in values. We doctors, often unknowingly, influence this process. We do because decisions on individual cases do have cumulative and declaratory effects. For instance, a pediatrician's decision to break an adolescent patient's confidential information about her sexual activity may add to the general concern among teenagers that doctors cannot be trusted to keep secrets.

The subject of medical advances relates closely to this topic. Whenever new treatments arise, public attention focuses on them and how doctors use them. A typical example occurred in 1981 when a Maryland physician prescribed estrogens to retarded adolescents who masturbated frequently. The intent was to diminish their sexual feelings and make them more available to interact with teachers and to alleviate the anxiety and apprehension of the surrounding adult caretakers. Yet, in spite of the good intentions, the fact remains that altering a normal biologic function as a solution to a troublesome behavior may subtly influence the attitude of society to behavioral problems in general.

We have to acknowledge that as physicians we are immersed in the ethical dimension. Sooner or later we cannot help but ask: what should be the pediatrician's involvement in moral education? Moral education is not, of course, the physician's primary responsibility but it is certainly not peripheral to pediatric practice. In our society moral education is not clearly defined. Family, schools, churches, and media all have a role to play; and frequently the doctor will become involved. Often when the question arises, "What ought to be done?" the pediatrician transcends his profession, and as a person, becomes a role model, a moral educator for better or for worse, whether he wants it or not. The pediatrician does not need to be a moralist, but he ought to be comfortable in his encounters with moral philosophy. From the time of Hippocrates this has been part of the physician's tradition. Our involvement is necessary; we should not forget that "the ultimate disease of our time is valuelessness."[11]

REFERENCES

1. Allen C: Textbook of Psychosexual Disorders. London, Oxford University Press, 1962.
2. Reich W: The Sexual Revolution. London, Vision Press, 1951.
3. Packard V: The Sexual Wilderness. New York, David McKay Co, 1968.
4. Inhelder B, Piaget J: The Growth of Logical Thinking from Childhood to Adolescence. New York, Basic Books, 1958.
5. Kohlberg L, Gilliam C: The adolescent as philosopher. Daedalus: Journal of the American Academy of Arts and Sciences, Fall 1971.
6. Silber TJ: The physician adolescent patient relationship. Clin Pediatr 19:50, 1980.
7. Committee on Adolescence, American Academy of Pediatrics: Contraception for the Adolescent. News and Comments, April 1980.
8. Silber TJ: Ethical considerations in the medical care of adolescents and their parents. Pediatr Ann 10:408, 1981.
9. Lemmon J: Moral Dilemmas. Philosophical Review, vol 71, 1962.
10. Oppenheimer C, Catalan J: Counseling for sexual problems. Ethical Issues and Decision Making. Practitioner 225:1623, 1981.
11. Maslow A: New Knowledge in Human Value. Henry Regner Co, New York, 1951.

Tomas J. Silber, M.D.

14

ETHICAL CONSIDERATIONS CONCERNING ADOLESCENTS CONSULTING FOR CONTRACEPTIVE SERVICES

More than 1 in 10 adolescent girls get pregnant every year. Four out of every 10 of them will get pregnant at least once during their teenage years. Seven million adolescent boys and five million adolescent girls are currently sexually active. One-fifth of teenage pregnancies occur in the first month of intercourse, and one-half of them occur in the first six months of sexual activity. The average teenager is sexually active a year or more before seeking contraceptive advice. One-third of those teenagers who consult for birth control say that their reason for delaying the medical visit was that they were afraid their families would find out.[1] The implications and consequences of adolescent pregnancy should be of grave concern to anybody working with teenagers.[2] This chapter addresses one particular and crucial concern: the ethical considerations involved in the medical care of adolescents who consult for contraceptive services.

THE PROBLEM

When an adolescent girl comes alone, or is brought in by her parents, to the physician's office for health assessment, she becomes the patient, and

Reprinted from the Journal of Family Practice, vol 15, no 5, 1982. Appleton-Century-Crofts, Publisher.

if responsibility is accepted for her care, the physician has an obligation to her.[3] How can the physician's obligation to the adolescent patient be reconciled with the physician's obligation to her parents? This problem may be best viewed in terms of consent and confidentiality.

CONSENT AND CONFIDENTIALITY

Consent is a contract between patient and physician. The physician must explain the nature of the treatment proposed as well as the existing alternatives, in return for which the patient will give permission to the physician for treatment. At this point a conflict emerges: In the case of the adolescent, neither a child nor an adult, who should give consent?

Confidentiality deals with the privileged nature of information provided to the physician by the adolescent. Accordingly, the medical history and the physical findings cannot be shared with others, including parents, without the adolescent's permission. Here a conflict arises: When adolescents who live at home engage in unprotected intercourse, which may place their health in danger and put them at high risk for pregnancy, should not the parents have a right to know?

The way in which the preceding questions are answered depends to some degree on how society defines children in relationship to their parents. Several approaches have been taken to answer these questions in a consistent fashion.[4]

Historically, the earliest response was to deny all rights to the adolescent. Adolescents therefore could not consent to their health care. Based on the concept of "parental sovereignty," parents assumed a claim of ownership of their children. This doctrine continues to be reflected in court rulings on custody, foster care, and adoption.

In the late nineteenth century, legal limits were imposed on parental ownership in those circumstances in which the children were considered to be in danger. This doctrine became known as the "child welfare" position and is clearly reflected by child abuse and compulsory education laws.[5]

In spite of their dissimilarity, both of these interpretations have a significant element in common: Adolescents have no rights of their own. Either the parent or the state determines what is to be in their best interest. A serious flaw of both the parental sovereignty doctrine and the child welfare doctrine is that neither distinguishes between the stages of complete dependency that characterize childhood and the autonomy that develops in adolescents. In the past two decades a new philosophy dealing with the issue of the "civil rights" of adolescents emerged, taking into account differences in age and maturity. This approach allows for parents or the state to represent the minors' interest only as long as such minors are not able to represent themselves.

A determining rule is proposed: The level of developmental capacity of the adolescent, rather than any arbitrary legal disposition, should be the deciding factor of competency for consent for treatment. Often referred to as the "mature minor doctrine," this concept is exemplified in recent legislation on freedom of speech in schools and the minor's right to obtain contraceptives. This pivotal idea has been expressed in the legal literature as follows: "A 'mature minor' does make his or her decisions on daily affairs, is mobile, independent, and can manage financial affairs; can initiate own appointments, understands risks, benefits, and informed consent (if anyone does!)."[6] The mature minor doctrine has been congruent with the viewpoint of specialists in child development and has been accepted by the American Academy of Pediatrics.[7] As a social definition it acknowledges the changes that come with the increasing cognitive competence of teenagers and affirms that they can make rational decisions and therefore are capable of giving informed consent.[8]

The ethical justification for this position is based on two principles: the principle of autonomy, which states that a person should have a say on any action that is going to affect him, and the principle of beneficence, which states that whenever something good can be done for a person, it should be done, or at least no barriers should be placed to attaining that good.

Applied to an adolescent who engages in unprotected intercourse, the principle of autonomy rejects the formulation that the adolescent is being protected when parental consent is requested as a prerequisite for medical care. Instead, it views the insistence on parental consent as a denial of the adolescent's rights as a person separate from his parents. The principle of beneficence clearly lends support to the mature minor doctrine. Many adolescents who need access to medical care in order to get contraceptive care would never consult a physician if the physician required parental consent prior to treatment. Under the same principle it is also easy to see how the confidentiality of the information given by the adolescent can be ethically justified. Lack of confidentiality would constitute a barrier to health care.

DISCUSSION

Some feel that parents have a right to complete information on the health condition of their children. Others fear that in advocating the acceptance of the adolescent's right to consent, too much power is given to the physician. All these concerns may be subsumed in another question: May an otherwise dependent adolescent be considered independent in relationship to contraception, especially since there are health risks associated with many contraceptive modalities?

Elimination of mandatory parental consent or mandatory parental notification does not imply that parental involvement is not important. Parental involvement is a recognized part of optimal health care for adolescents.[9] The physician in reality is not in an adversary position toward the parent when he obtains the adolescent's consent and maintains the confidentiality in the relationship (although parents might not perceive it this way). The physician shares the same goal with the adolescent's family: to protect and restore the adolescent's health.

Physicians do encourage their adolescent patients to seek support from their families; they often act as an intermediary during a crisis, and they help to restore the organization of the family they care for. There is also no question that physicians value life above confidentiality and that they will breach confidentiality in cases of dangerous behavior, such as an adolescent's refusal to be hospitalized if she suffers from a complication stemming from the use of a contraceptive method. However, whenever such an unusual step must be taken, it is the physician's obligation to inform the patient about the breach of confidentiality and the rationale for it.

The legal implications of ethical considerations such as these become a matter of state law. Most states have laws establishing that minors may give consent for their treatment under specified conditions. Suspicion of pregnancy qualifies in most state legislations. In addition, there are laws that go even further, creating the category of "emancipated minor." Courts determining who fits this category take into account such conditions as "living apart from parents," "having a child," "being a member of the armed forces," and so on, and such criteria vary from state to state. The principle has been tested in the case of a 17-year-old girl who had consented to medical treatment without her parents' knowledge.[10] In spite of good medical results, the parents sued the physician on the reasoning that because their daughter was a minor, she could not give consent for treatment and had therefore been treated without valid consent. They lost. The trial court held that the state law insulated the treating physician from liability, a ruling that was subsequently affirmed on appeal.

From the viewpoint of malpractice liability, at present physicians are required to know the condition and circumstances under which their states allow them to treat adolescents without parental consent as well as what constitutes an "emancipated minor" in their jurisdiction. If consultation about possible pregnancy or contraception is not covered by the state law, the physician must determine if the patient fits the "emancipated minor" status. This determination should be documented in the medical record. It is of interest to note that many state laws provide that physicians and health care facilities cannot be held liable for accepting a minor's consent in good faith. Thus, misrepresentation by a minor regarding, for example, the degree of his independence will not invalidate the consent accepted in good faith by the treating physician.

The debate on the adolescent's right to consent and confidentiality is only one component of a larger struggle in moral philosophy. This society stands at the crossroads of a number of different ethical systems. Each is the carrier of a highly particular kind of moral tradition, as evidenced by "parental sovereignty," "child welfare," and "adolescent rights." Of course, when such moral traditions encounter each other, they are to some degree damaged and fragmented in the process. Thus, it comes as no surprise that the confusions of pluralism are often expressed in issues that relate to the status of adolescents. Though this confusion is being clarified through guidelines and by statutory regulations, conscientious reflection by physicians is necessary concerning the nature of their commitments to adolescents and their parents.

SUMMARY

Adolescents increasingly come to physicians' offices for contraceptive care. This raises the issue of parental involvement, often formulated in terms of conflict around the issues of consent and confidentiality. In the past two decades, a new philosophy has emerged that deals with the issues from a perspective of the "civil rights" of adolescents. This concept, referred to as the "mature minor doctrine," allows for parents or the state to represent the minors' interest only as long as the adolescent is not able to do so. The ethical justification for this position is based on the principles of autonomy and beneficence. The legal implications are being developed in state laws which recognize that teenagers should have access to confidential medical care in order to facilitate contraceptive knowledge and prevention of pregnancy.

REFERENCES

1. Teenage Pregnancy: The Problem that Hasn't Gone Away. New York, Alan Guttmacher Institute, 1981.
2. Silber T: Adolescent pregnancy: A new perspective. Clin Proc 36:350, 1980.
3. Silber T: The physician-adolescent patient relationship. Clin Pediatr 19:50, 1980.
4. Hofmann A: A rational policy toward consent and confidentiality in adolescent health care. J Adol Health Care 1:9, 1980.
5. Goldstein J, Freud A, Solnit A: Beyond the Best Interest of the Child. New York, The Free Press, 1980.
6. Brown RH, Truitt RB: Right of minors to medical treatment. DePaul Law Review 28:290, 1979.
7. American Academy of Pediatrics: A model act providing for consent of minors for health services. Pediatrics 51:293, 1973.
8. Inhelder B, Piaget J: The Growth of Logical Thinking From Childhood to Adolescence. New York, Basic Books, 1958.
9. Committee on Adolescence: Health Assessment and Health Maintenance for the Adolescent. Evanston, Ill, American Academy of Pediatrics, 1980.
10. *Carter v Cangello*, 165 Cal Rptr 363 (Cal App May 1, 1980).

Special Problems

1. Beauchamp TL, Walters L (eds): Contemporary Issues in Bioethics. Encino, CA, Dickenson Publishing Co., 1978.
2. Brody H: Placebos and the Philosophy of Medicine: Clinical, Conceptual and Ethical Issues. Chicago, The University of Chicago Press, 1980.
3. Munson R: Intervention and Reflection: Basic Issues in Medical Ethics. Belmont, CA, Wadsworth Publishing Co., 1979.
4. Robison, WL, Pritchard MS (eds): Medical Responsibility. Clifton, NJ, Humana Press, 1979.
5. Singer P: Practical Ethics. Cambridge, Cambridge University Press, 1979.
6. Veatch RM: Case Studies in Medical Ethics. Cambridge, MA, Harvard University Press, 1977.

SECTION FIVE

EXPERIMENTATION WITH CHILDREN

The scientific justification for including children in biomedical research is that their physiology and development is unique and therefore cannot be replaced by another model. However, there remain moral questions about the legitimacy of their participation in research, both therapeutic and nontherapeutic, and the rights of parents to give consent in the name of their children. In the early 1970s, Ramsey tackled this issue, opposing any nontherapeutic research on children. This argument was based on the concept that nontherapeutic research should never be performed without the informed consent of the research subject. Since young children are incapable of giving formal consent, no research should be performed. In response to this position, McCormick developed a less restrictive position based on the acceptance of the risks of nontherapeutic research whenever they are minimal and the potential benefits of the research are great. Under such circumstances, experimentation with parental consent would be morally justified. The intense controversy on this issue finally resulted in a collective work, drafted by the National Commission for the Protection of Human Subjects of Biomedical and Behavioral Research, the Report and Recommendation on Research Involving Children. Albert Jonsen presents a clear exposition of these recommendations. Angela Holder completes this section, elaborating on the concept of when an adolescent may participate in research based on his own consent.

Albert R. Jonsen, Ph.D.

15

RESEARCH INVOLVING CHILDREN

Throughout history, children have been subjects of research. A legendary Persian prince is said to have isolated newborn babies from all human speech in hopes of discovering whether language was natural and spontaneous. Queen Caroline of England recruited children from a foundling hospital in order to test Jenner's vaccination on them before it was applied to her own royal progeny. The modern controversy over research with children and the retarded can be traced to events at Willowbrook State Hospital for the Mentally Retarded where, during the 1950s and 1960s, healthy mentally retarded children were infected with mild hepatitis in order to study the natural history of the disease. That research aroused great public controversy, and its merits and faults are debated even today. It initiated a discussion within and without the medical profession over whether any invasion or manipulation of the body or person of a nonconsenting subject could ever be ethically justified, apart from expectation of benefit to that subject.[1]

The prevailing codes of ethics governing the use of human subjects for experimentation are curiously ambivalent about children. The progenitor of these codes, The Code of Nuremberg, if taken literally, would exclude children as subjects, for it requires the voluntary consent of the subject "as absolutely essential," without any provision for proxy consent.[2] The World

Reprinted by courtesy of Pediatrics 62:131–136, 1978.

Medical Association's Declaration of Helsinki, on the other hand, states that for nontherapeutic research involving legally incompetent subjects, "the consent of the legal guardian should be procured."[3] This position has been adopted by the American Medical Association:

> Minors or mentally incompetent persons may be used as subjects only if (i) the nature of the investigation is such that mentally competent adults would not be suitable subjects: (ii) consent, in writing, is given by a legally authorized representative of the subject under circumstances in which an informed and prudent adult would reasonably be expected to volunteer himself or his child as a subject.

This position, permitting nontherapeutic research on the basis of proxy consent of the legally authorized representative, was tacitly accepted by the U.S. Department of Health, Education, and Welfare.[4]

It is not an unchallenged position. Beecher cited (and disagreed with) the purported British position that any medical intervention on a normal child, or on a sick child without the intent to provide therapy, was ethically and legally unacceptable.[5] A case currently sub judice seeks to establish this position in an American jurisdiction, arguing that parents have no legal right to consent to any intervention on their child that is not directed at the child's benefit.[6] The philosophers and theologians continue to debate the question, Princeton's Paul Ramsey and Georgetown's Richard McCormick taking opposing views. The former repudiates any ethical justification for research with a normal child; the latter claims that even children bear a certain obligation to benefit society that justifies a presumption of their consent to experiments of minimal risk.[7,8]

At the heart of the legal and ethical controversy are two central issues: (1) proxy consent and (2) the relevance of risk-benefit assessment. The National Commission for the Protection of Human Subjects of Biomedical and Behavioral Research, established by Congress in 1974, has been charged with an investigation of these issues, with regard to research involving children and the institutionalized mentally incompetent.[9] I have been a member of this Commission since its inception. The Commission has completed its recommendations on these issues. These recommendations will doubtless influence federal policy governing the conduct and support of research involving children. These recommendations, which are the result of extensive review of the problems of research with children, suggest new avenues of thinking about the ethics of research with children. They should help resolve some hitherto paradoxic questions; they will also create new paradoxes. These recommendations of the National Commission have been presented to the Secretary of DHEW. He is required by law to publish these recommendations in the *Federal Register* and, following comment from the interested public, to issue regulations. The law that established the Commission orders the Secretary to offer reasons, should his final regulations depart in any significant way from the recommendations of the Commission. The recommendations have appeared in the *Federal Register* (January 13,

1978) and are open to comments that should be directed to the Secretary of DHEW.[10]

In the remainder of this chapter I set out in summary form the ten recommendations of the Commission and the deliberations that led to them. It is not my intent to defend at length those points which are certain to be controversial, but merely to expose the results of the Commission's deliberations to the community of those involved in the care of children. While I will attempt to be faithful to the recommendations and deliberations in this summary, I may, as I paraphrase them, show my own interpretations. Thus, I must assert that I speak here only for myself and not as a spokesperson for my fellow commissioners.

THE RECOMMENDATIONS

The Commission defines "children" as "individuals who have not attained the age of consent for medical care or for research activities in the jurisdiction in which the research will be conducted." The Commission defines "research activities" as all procedures performed in a "formal investigation designed to contribute to generalizable knowledge." They include, but are not limited to, diagnostic, prophylactic, and therapeutic interventions that are the focus of systematic investigation, and other interventions or modifications of procedures, observations, comparisons, measurements, the use of questionnaires and surveys, and the analysis of data, undertaken for the purpose of obtaining specific information.

The first recommendation is a general commendation of research involving children. It expresses the findings that research is valuable and necessary for the health and well-being of children, that it can be done ethically, and that it should be supported by the Secretary of DHEW under the specific conditions set forth in the following nine recommendations.[11] This is not an empty accolade for research; it is based on a survey of the nature and extent of current research supported by the federal government, on a staff report stating the scientific reasons in favor of research involving children, and on the testimony of leaders from the pediatric research community. The opinion that this research can be done in an ethical manner rests on a survey of institutional review boards, arguments presented by experts in law and ethics, and testimony from those concerned about the welfare of children. All this evidence is presented in summary in the Commission's report and recommendations and are published in full in the appendix to the report.

The second recommendation states the general conditions that must be fulfilled in order for any proposed research to be judged ethical. The institutional review board (required by 1966 DHEW guidelines in all institutions where DHEW funds support research) must determine several points. First, the research must be scientifically sound and significant; studies must first be performed in animals and adults, and in older children before infants, if this is possible; risks must be minimized by using the safest procedures consistent with research design; privacy and confidentiality must be protected, and subjects must be selected in an equitable manner. Researchers should avail themselves of indicated diagnostic and therapeutic procedures for research purposes whenever this is feasible. In addition, the permission of parents and the assent of children, when they are capable, must be obtained. Particulars concerning parental permission and assent of children are stated in recommendations 7 throught 10.[11]

Recommendation 3 states that "research that does not involve greater than minimal risk to children" may be conducted, provided that all the conditions of recommendation 2 are met and the requirements for permission and assent have been fulfilled.[11] In its definitions, the Commission stipulates that "minimal risk" should be taken to mean "the probability and magnitude of physical or psychological harm that is normally encountered in the daily lives, or in the routine medical or psychological examination of healthy children."[11] It offers as examples immunization, modest changes in diet or schedule, physical and developmental examinations, and the obtaining of blood and urine specimens. The possible effects of disruption of normal routine, separation from parents, or unusual discomfort should be considered, as well as the more obvious risks. The measure of minimal risk in research is, in general, the sort of risk that normal children run in the course of their daily lives. This is, of course, a very conservative norm. Nevertheless, in allowing even this, the Commission takes a position contrary to some ethical and legal commentators.[5-7] It takes this position because its deliberations led to the conclusion that profound parental concern for the welfare of children was not incompatible with allowing children to enter situations that entail minimal risks. Indeed, this seems to be so in the course of daily life and may even be thought of as the education intrinsic to living in the world. Further, the Commission has noted that much of the research involving children involves nothing more than observation and measurements, in which the research as such presents no discernible risks.

Recommendation 4 turns to the problem of research in which the risks would be "more than minimal." The Commission allows such research when the intervention holds out the prospect of direct benefit for the individual subject. Greater risks can be tolerated when, for example, all available treatments for a disorder have been exhausted and a procedure under investigation for safety and efficacy is available, or when a new procedure appears to be more efficacious or less dangerous than a standard one. The procedure under investigation must have a ratio of anticipated benefit to risk at least as favorable as other treatment alternatives, as well as the alternative of providing no treatment at all.[11]

In this recommendation, the Commisison has endorsed the long-accepted principle that whenever benefit and harm may accrue to the same person, and when that person is in need of assistance, it is ethical to proceed if it can be shown that the expected benefits "outweigh" the risks. It is obvious that "weighing" is not a quantitative activity, although statistic data about risks and benefits might be helpful. Rather, the acceptability of benefits and

risks is a matter of discretion; parents, researchers, therapists, reviewers, and, in some circumstances, the child must judge.

Recommendations 5 and 6 address the most difficult problem raised by research involving children: Is it ethical to expose a child to risks that are more than minimal when the interventions dictated solely for research purposes are not intended to benefit the individual subject? The first instinct of the commissioners was, I believe, that such a situation could not be tolerated. As one commissioner said on viewing an early version of this recommendation, "utterly delete it." However, on reflection, an absolute prohibition on "nonbeneficial and more than minimal risk" activities seemed unreasonable. Many children suffer from debilitating disorders and fatal diseases whose etiology is poorly understood and for which there are no or, at best, inadequate therapies. Studies performed on these children could advance the understanding of the disease and might lead to the development and improvement of therapies. The affected children themselves may be the only sources of that information. On the other hand, the prospects of an effective therapy might be so remote that barring a breakthrough, they may never be beneficiaries of improved understanding of their condition. Indeed, it may be wholly unlikely that they could be helped, as in the case of most mental disability or many neurologic disorders; still, the condition from which they suffer incurably might be prevented in the future. Given such situations, would it be ethical to do studies that might entail more than minimal risk to these children?

The Commission faced the cruel dilemma: either protect children from any research risk that is more than minimal, and thereby prevent the possible discovery of means to cure or prevent certain serious disorders, or, by endangering some children, seek the well-being of future ones. Some philosophers will assert that this is not in fact a dilemma, since there is no positive duty to benefit, while there is a duty to prevent harm. Yet, to many, this philosophic consideration seems to be an abstract and heartless solution. On the other hand, the Commission was not satisfied with the argument often advanced by researchers: the prospect of great future good overrides the dangers imposed on a few present subjects. Between these positions, the Commission chose a middle path that seemed reasonable and ethically defensible to all its members except two, who dissented over recommendation 5.

The recommendation, then, allows that children might be entered into research entailing more than minimal risk and promising no individual benefit when (1) the risk entailed represents "a minor increase over minimal risk," (2) the experience presented by the intervention is "reasonably commensurate with those inherent in the actual or expected medical, psychological or social situation" of the subject, and (3) the research is likely to yield generalizable knowledge about the subject's condition that is "of vital importance for understanding and amelioration of the condition" from which that class of subjects suffers. Finally, all provisions regarding permission and assent must be met.[11]

In this recommendation, the Commission offers two important and equally necessary considerations about risks in this sort of research. First, it states that any additional risks must represent but a minor increase over minimal risk. While the actual determination of risk remains a matter for prudent discretion, the rule of "no more than minimal risk," defined as the ordinary risks of childhood, remains the standard for judgment. "Minor increase" over minimal risk refers to risks of harm or discomforts greater in probability and magnitude than those encountered in the normal life of children but that pose no significant threat to the child's well-being. Thus, a biopsy, a spinal tap, or the dose of an acceptable level of a radioisotope, while surpassing the risks of daily life, are unlikely to cause any serious harm. Second, these risks must be "reasonably commensurate with the subject's own experiences." The children envisioned in these recommendations will be children who, because of their illness, will be subject to frequent diagnostic, palliative, and therapeutic interventions. In the course of their care, they will undergo certain painful, uncomfortable, or risky interventions. The Commission suggests that any research procedures resemble, in ways that the children can identify, the experiences with which they are familiar. This does not, of course, refer to the magnitude and the probability of the occurrence of harm, which, if assimilated to many diagnostic and therapeutic risks, would be unacceptable. It refers rather to actual experience of the intervention. Thus, a request for a spinal tap for research purposes alone may be "reasonably commensurate" for a child under treatment for hydrocephalus. Should the child be capable of assent, "commensurability" should aid that child to understand the procedure by giving some standard for comparison and to determine whether he or she wishes to participate when it is explained that this intervention is not necessary for his or her care. Should the child be unable to assent, "commensurability" should assist parents to comprehend the nature of the research procedure and ability of their child to tolerate it.

The requirement of commensurability is not intended to give researchers unlimited access to sick children. It must be seen in conjunction with the other elements of this recommendation: the children involved must be the sole source of relevant information, the information must be "of vital importance," and any additional risks must be, at most, "minor" increments over minimal. Within such a research design, the research must constitute an experience that while possibly unpleasant, is not foreign to the child. Commensurability is intended to enhance the child's understanding and tolerance of the research procedure—not to add to its riskiness. Several commissioners dissented from this recommendation. One judged that this criterion would be misused to the disadvantage of sick children; the other felt that allowing minor increment over minimal risks gave too much discretion to local review boards.[11]

Recommendation 6 states that should an institutional review board be unable to approve research under the previous recommendations and, at the same time, estimate that the research presents an "opportunity to understand, prevent or alleviate a serious problem affecting the health or welfare of children," the board may send the protocol on for review by a national ethical advisory board. Presumably, this would arise when there are serious unanswered questions about the magnitude of risk, the likelihood of benefit, and the importance of the problem. Should the testing of the polio vaccine in children be proposed today, the process of coming to a decision would follow the path laid down by this recommendation. In addition, it appeared to the Commission that the probability of exposure of any citizen to serious risks for the public good raised problems of public policy far beyond the scope of review by boards and regulations by agencies. This is a public issue of magnitude, and thus any determination by a national review board should be open to review by the Congress. The reason for this is stated by Commissioner Louisell in his comment on the previous recommendation: "Such experimentation on children can be morally justified, if even ever, only to fulfill an essential social need analogous to that involved in the drafting of youth for national security purposes. Resolution of this kind of a moral dilemma in a democracy at a minimum requires decision by society's highest political voice."[11]

In recommendations 2 through 6, the Commission responds to its mandate to study the role of risk-benefit criteria. In recommendations 7 through 10, it addresses its other principal mandate, a study of the problem of informed consent. These two issues are complementary: every proposed protocol for research must be judged both in terms of risk-benefit assessment and in terms of consent. In the case of children, it is clear that their own "voluntary participation" is sometimes quite impossible and is always limited. On the other hand, questions have been raised about the propriety and adequacy of any proxy consent by parents or guardians. After seeking the views of lawyers, ethicists, and professionals who deal with children, the Commission debated these problems at length. Recommendation 7 states its basic position:

> The institutional review board should determine that adequate provisions are made for: (A) soliciting the assent of the children (when capable) and the permission of their parents or guardians and monitoring this process (when appropriate); and (B) involving at least one parent or guardian in the conduct of research when the prospective subjects are infants and a significant departure from normal routine or more than minimal risk is presented.[11]

The Commission requires the institutional review board to ascertain whether children whose participation is sought live within strong, protective familial settings and whether the family has made a "collective judgment" about the entry of the child. If the children are infants, the institutional review board may recommend or require the actual presence of parents at the time of the research procedure.

The Commission's position on this point was determined by its view of the parental role. The traditional opinion that parents may give proxy consent for experimentation seemed unsatisfactory. First, it is clear that the child is not, himself, consenting. Although some theory about what the child "would do" or "ought to do" might be constructed, it is best to acknowledge frankly the fact that the child does nothing that can be called "consenting." Second, having admitted this, it seemed that parental authority was based on profound concern and involvement of parents for their children. Proxy consent seemed too remote and too legalistic a term to describe this. Thus, the Commission felt that more than minimal-risk research could be tolerated only if the parents were seriously engaged in the judgment about the child's participation and, indeed, even participated themselves in some way in the experimental procedure. On certain occasions, their presence at the time of the experimental procedures might be required by the board for the reassurance of the child. Considerable discretion is allowed to institutional review boards in making these determinations, but researchers are encouraged to design research in ways that meet these standards. Behind the recommendations, which may appear strange and difficult to fulfill, lies the conviction that a high degree of parental involvement and the deliberate careful reduction of any risks entailed in the research are concomitant requisites of any ethical decision to allow children to be entered in research. This conviction closely mirrors the parental responsibility for the normal welfare, life, growth, and health of their children.

The Commission also requires that the assent of children be sought when possible. The word "assent" is chosen to distinguish the child's agreement from a legally valid consent, and to recognize that it is more limited than the consent of adults. Children mature in their ability to understand and to engage themselves in various activities. The Commission believes that the ethical principle of respect urges acknowledgment of that developing ability. It suggests, somewhat arbitrarily but still on the basis of common experience, that the age of seven may be an appropriate time to begin requiring parents and investigators to seek the child's assent. A child's objection to participation should be binding, unless the research promises direct benefit that is available only in the context of research; for example, when the use of an experimental drug seems to be indicated for therapeutic purposes.

Recommendation 8 acknowledges that parental consent may not always be a protection for the child. Certain research, such as the study of social conditions leading to teenage sexual activity or of the use of contraceptives by teenagers, may be informative and useful in alleviating personal and social problems. Many jurisdictions allow minors to seek medical care in these matters without parental permission. It seems reasonable, then, to allow the board to waive parental permission in such circumstances, provided an adequate mechanism for the protection of children is devised, such as the appointment of a noninvolved person particularly devoted to the welfare of children and skilled in dealing with them as a special advisor to, and advocate for, the young potential subject.[11] Recommendation 9 prohibits the inclusion of wards of the state in research unless the research is related to their status as orphan or abandoned children. Such children, by definition, lack the strong familial protection that the Commission desires as the usual condition for participation. If any research involving these children is approved, each child should be assigned an advocate.[11] Recommendation 10 simply calls attention to the fact that the Commission has made particular recommendations to cover the special problems of research in correctional institutions and in institutions for the mentally infirm. Any research involving children in such places must conform to these recommendations as well as the present ones.[11]

I found the devising of these recommendations to be an extremely difficult task. I believe my colleagues on the Commission would all agree. At almost every point, we found ourselves confronted by paradoxes, turning usually on conflict between two important values: the protection of children and the improvement of their care. Very strong arguments were offered, both by our consultants and by the commissioners, on both sides of each contentious point. Often, even the strongest arguments left the issues unresolved in any intellectually satisfactory way. Yet, we were required to develop some public policy that would be reasonable, enforceable, and in conformity with fundamental moral beliefs of our culture.

The recommendations may not satisfy these criteria. They may draw many criticisms from many sources. However, they do represent the considered conclusions of the most serious and extensive deliberations that have ever taken place on this delicate problem.

REFERENCES

1. Katz J: Experimentation With Human Beings. New York, Russell Sage Foundation, 1972, pp 1007–1010.
2. Trials of War Criminals Before the Nuremberg Military Tribunals: United States v. Karl Brandt. US Government Printing Office, 1949, vol 2, p 181.
3. World Medical Association: Declaration of Helsinki, 1964. *In* Beecher H (ed): Research and the Individual: Human Studies. Boston, Little Brown & Co, 1970.
4. The Institutional Guide to DHEW Policy on Protection of Human Subjects, DHEW publication (NIH) 72-102. US Dept of Health, Education and Welfare, Dec 1, 1971, p 71.
5. Medical Research Council, Great Britain: Responsibility in investigations on human subjects. *In* Beecher H (ed): Research and the Individual: Human Subjects. Boston, Little Brown & Co, 1970, pp 262–265.
6. Nielson v. Regents of University of California. Civil No. 665-049, California Supreme Count, Dec 19, 1973.
7. Ramsey P: The enforcement of morals: Nontherapeutic research on children. Hastings Center Rep, August 1976, pp 21–30.
8. McCormick R: Proxy consent in the experimental situation. Perspect Biol Med 18:2, 1974.
9. Public law 93:348, July 12, 1974.
10. Federal Register 43:2084 (Jan 13) 1978.
11. National Commission for the Protection of Human Subjects of Biomedical and Behavioral Research: Report and Recommendations on Research Involving Children, DHEW publication (05)77-0004. US Dept of Health, Education and Welfare, 1977.

Angela R. Holder, L.L.M.

16

CAN TEENAGERS PARTICIPATE IN RESEARCH WITHOUT PARENTAL CONSENT?

- An investigator at a university medical school posted notices recruiting subjects for venipuncture. Payment will be $5.00. A 16-year-old freshman in the college sees one of the posters and wishes to participate.
- An investigator wants to survey attitudes about abortion in a group of 16-year-olds who have had first-trimester abortions. These young women are now patients in a family planning clinic, and their parents do not know about their abortions or that they are now receiving contraceptives.
- A political scientist wants to survey a variety of people in the community, from junior high school students to senior citizens, to find out what percentage approve of the guarantees in the Bill of Rights or even recognize it when they see a copy. One group he wants to include is 16-year-old volunteers at a day-care center, all of whom are taking a required high school civics course.
- A physician wishes to treat with an investigational drug a 16-year-old patient whose leukemia is not responding to standard therapy.

Reprinted with permission of The Hastings Center, Institute of Society, Ethics and the Life Sciences, 360 Broadway, Hastings-on-Hudson, NY 10706.

Which, if any, of these 16-year-olds may legally consent to participate in research without parental permission?

An adolescent's legal capacity to consent to participation in research is usually discussed in the context of consent to medical treatment. While this is probably the closest legal analogy with which investigators and IRB members are familiar, much of the research aimed at the teenage population is not related to biomedical research at all. Probably most of those who want to dispense with parental permission are not medical researchers but social scientists who want to administer questionnaires, surveys, and various education tests to adolescents. School administrators made this point in responding to the National Commission for the Protection of Human Subjects' recommendations for regulating research on children by urging DHEW to exempt from parental-consent requirements all educational research, even on primary-grade students, conducted in schools.[1] The legal-medical model is, however, the basic framework in which most cases involving these issues have been adjudicated.

In the past decade legislatures and courts have been increasingly willing to expand adolescents' rights to consent to reasonable medical intervention, and many physicians seem unaware of the degree to which teenagers are now regarded as legally autonomous. In common law, a child (which included anyone under 21), was, in effect, a chattel of his or her parents with virtually no legal protection against their decisions. Child abuse, for example, did not become a crime until very late in the nineteenth century. Children were regarded as economic benefits to their parents, and courts viewed any threat to their utility value with strong disapproval. Although medical treatment could be given without parental consent in life-threatening emergencies, nonemergency medical interventions, even if the results were entirely successful, provided without parental consent gave the parents (not the child) a cause of action against the physician. The legal theory was that the parents could recover damages from the physician for interference with their rights to custody and control.

The doctrine of emancipation developed as a means of enforcing contractual obligations undertaken by young men in their late teens (women's capacity at the time to contract at any age being severely limited), and eventually the courts regarded the independent minor as an adult. The minor in military service was clearly emancipated and, among other things, could consent to medical care, since it was somewhat impractical to get permission from a soldier's mother or father to treat battlefield injuries.[2] Married minors were also emancipated, thus freeing their parents from any further duty of support. Most self-supporting minors who were living away from home were considered "emancipated," at least by the mid-1920s. Most states now have statutes defining emancipation; while these vary considerably, in most states, for example, a college student less than 18 living in a dormitory is normally considered to be emancipated, even if entirely supported by his or her parents. Motherhood is now considered evidence of emancipation, regardless of chronologic age, at least for purposes of consenting to medical care for one's self and one's baby or for surrendering the baby for adoption. In many states, a teenage mother is emancipated for all purposes.

In addition to liberalization of the concept of emancipation, beginning in the 1950s all states enacted statutes specifically permitting a minor of any age to consent to treatment for venereal disease (VD) without parental knowledge. If notification of parents was a precondition of treatment, of course, the teenager would very likely forego therapy rather than have parents find out it was necessary, thus further spreading the "epidemic" of VD in young people. Most states have also recently developed analogous statutes to include treatment for alcohol and drug abuse. Beyond statutory authority for treatment of these specific conditions, a majority of states provide a specific statutory age (usually 15 or 16, but 14 in at least one state) at which a minor may consent to any medical or surgical care without parental involvement.[3]

Even where there is no such statute and the minor is not emancipated, however, not a single case has been reported in this country in at least 15 years in which a parent recovered damages from a physician for treating a person of 15 years of age or older without parental consent. If the treatment was appropriate and no claim of malpractice is raised, and the teenaged patient was as capable of giving an informed consent as an adult, courts have allowed that consent to prevail over parental objections raised after the fact. This trend in case law is known as "the mature minor rule."[4] By contrast, a parent's consent is still necessary for nonemergency treatment of a younger child; and courts have made clear that parents have the right to refuse to allow elective medical interventions.[5] A teenager, as well as an adult, also has a constitutional right of privacy in some circumstances involving medical care. The Supreme Court has held that parents have no veto over their daughter's decision to have an abortion, although commentators disagree on the extent to which the Supreme Court decisions abrogate the daughter's right to privacy in terms of parental notification if a state statute requires it.[6] The Court has also held that minors do have a right of privacy in obtaining contraception.[7]

Research involving surveys or questionnaires, particularly if conducted in schools, may also raise privacy issues. In responding to school administrators' comments that parental consent should not be required for educational testing, DHEW indicated that it would be bound by the precedent established in the case of *Merriken v. Cressman*.[8] A school board attempted to implement a program of required "psychologic testing" of junior high school students to discover "deviant" personalities who would be likely to become involved with drugs. Those whose scores put them in the "deviant" group would be put in special classes and their "deviancy" classification circulated widely to teachers, coaches, and counselors. No parental permission was sought. If the student objected to the test, including questions about whether he or she had been hugged when small and other extremely personal questions about the family, there was an automatic score of "deviance." A 13-year-old eighth-grader refused to take the test, and he and his mother asked the court to stop the testing. The court ruled that since the boy had no right to refuse and the test score would be placed on his permanent record, his right of privacy had been violated. The court noted that his mother had not been asked to consent, but that issue was quite secondary to the violation of the student's privacy right. This case is not a useful guide, however, because it did not involve a research project, and the court did not discuss whether such a test would have been permissible if the students had been able to give a noncoerced consent.

In making analogies to the medical model, it is now clear that adolescents do have extensive freedom to consent to therapeutic interventions, even to those carrying substantial risks. If the parents are unavailable or the teenager refuses to discuss the situation with them, a physician is undoubtedly legally protected, at least short of high-risk surgery, if treatment is undertaken on the basis of the adolescent's informed consent. However, one basic limitation is imposed by factors having little to do with the adolescent's legal rights: a parent is not financially responsible for nonemergency medical treatment that is provided without his or her knowledge.[9] Since few unemancipated minors, who by definition are not self-supporting, have their own financial resources for major medical interventions or protracted medical care, the teenager's access to, for example, cosmetic surgery requiring in-patient hospitalization without disclosure to parents is tempered by the physician's and hospital's willingness to provide free or low-cost care. Thus, the liberality of current law that would, for example, permit 16-year-olds to consent to rhinoplasty without their parents' knowledge has probably not resulted in many such operations.

On the other hand, if an intervention carries substantial risks and is for the primary benefit of someone other than the adolescent—for example, donation of a kidney to a sibling—even parental consent as well as the adolescent's is insufficient. A court order is required.[10] The difference, however, appears not to be so much the presence or absence of benefit as the presence or absence of an acceptable risk-benefit ratio. Where there is no benefit to the particular minor, there must also be no risk. For example, although the Red Cross requires blood donors to be 18 or older, probably to avoid the administrative inconvenience of establishing national guidelines for accepting "mature" minors but not others, it is highly improbable that a court would hold, if asked to rule on the question, that parental rights were violated by donation of a pint of blood or that the doctrine of *parens patriae* required a court order before a blood donation could be made.

The Commission's Report and Recommendations for Research on Children specifically attempted to deal with this problem on a common-sense basis.[11] Recommendation 8 provides:

> If the Institutional Review Board determines that a research protocol is designed for conditions or a subject population for which parental or guardian permission is not a reasonable requirement to protect the subjects, it may waive such requirement provided an appropriate mechanism for protecting the children who will participate as subjects in the research is substituted. The choice

of an appropriate mechanism should depend upon the nature and purpose of the activities described in the protocol, the risk and anticipated benefit to the research subjects, and their age, status and condition.

If this recommendation is incorporated into a regulation, it would dispense with the necessity of parental permission for participation in research equivalent to most treatment interventions for which the adolescent may now consent—as long as the local IRB felt that requiring permission would be "unreasonable." It is unlikely, as a practical matter, that an IRB will be inclined to allow waiver of parental permission in any research involving more than minimal risk of physical harm.

Investigators who deal with adolescent subjects are, in general, doing one of four sorts of research:

1. Adolescence is relevant to the condition studied—for example, the survey of young women's responses to having had abortions. In this context, not only would it be an imposition on a teenager whose parents do not already know about her abortion to get their permission to participate, she would undoubtedly simply decline to be surveyed. Thus, it would be impossible to obtain valuable information about such aspects of the problem as what sort of emotional support is available to adolescents who do not confide in their families about abortion. It would seem appropriate not to require parental consent in these situations.

2. Adolescence is irrelevant to the research—the volunteer for venipuncture. Most IRBs would usually waive parental permission only where there is little or no risk involved, and of course there is very substantial doubt that a healthy minor may participate in research involving any serious risk, even with parental permission.[12] Thus, the adolescent in the case should be able to participate.

3. The research involves an attempt to recruit subjects from various age groups—the political scientist's survey about the Bill of Rights. There may be some doubt that students have a genuine right to refuse to participate in research conducted in their high school classrooms, since the situation may be inherently coercive. Particularly in cases where any sensitive information contained in the research results might be identifiable and could find its way into the student's school records, an IRB might wish to require parental permission. If the information is, as in this example, not particularly sensitive and the survey is not conducted in a school, however, there seems to be no reason to require parental notification or consent.

4. The biomedical research is not related to the patient's age, but an adolescent patient has a disease the investigator wishes to study or an investigational drug is proposed for treatment—the patient with leukemia. Since investigational therapy with a risk of serious side effects is reserved for conditions that are themselves serious, regardless of the patient/subject's age, it is not very likely that the adolescent's treatment is being undertaken without parental knowledge unless the minor is emancipated in the strictest construction of the term—married or in military service. The possibility that

physician would agree to treat an unemancipated teenager for leukemia or other life-threatening illness without involving his or her parents in the first place, long before the issue of investigational therapy arises, is extremely remote.

Thus, protocols of this sort are quite unlikely to present the issue of waiver of parental permission. If they do, however, parental permission probably should be required.

DHHS's proposed regulations for research on children appear to incorporate the Commission's view, as do the FDA proposals.[13,14] If the IRB determines that a protocol is designed "for conditions or for a subject population for which parental permission is not a reasonable requirement," it may waive the requirement. Unfortunately, however, the examples cited in the discussions of both sets of proposals are "neglected or abused children." These children present entirely different problems from self-reliant adolescents, and it is quite possible that IRB members may not realize from reading the proposed regulations that parental permission may be unnecessary in the sorts of situations under discussion.

REFERENCES

1. 43 *Fed. Reg.* 31786-31794, July 21, 1978, p. 31791.
2. *Swenson v. Swenson*, 227 SW 2d 103, Mo., 1950.
3. A state-by-state table of statutes involving minors' capacity to consent to medical care may be found in The National Commission for the Protection of Human Subjects of Biomedical and Behavioral Research: Report and Recommendations: Research Involving Children. DHEW Publication No. (OS) 77-0004, Washington, 1977.
4. Wadlington W: Minors and health care: The age of consent. Osgood Hall Law J. 11:115, 1973.
5. *In re Hudson*, 126 P 2d 765, Wash., 1942; *In re Seiferth*, 127 NE 2d 820, N.Y., 1955; *In re Tuttendario*, 21 Pa. Dist. 562, Pa., 1912.
6. *Bellotti v. Baird*, 443 U.S. 622, 1979; *Planned Parenthood v. Danforth*, 428 U.S. 952, 1976.
7. *Carey v. Population Services International*, 431 U.S. 678, 1977.
8. *Merriken v. Cressman*, 364 F. Supp. 913, DC Pa., 1973.
9. *Poudre Valley Hospital District v. Heckart*, 491 P 2d 984, Colo., 1971; *Ison v. Florida Sanitarium and Benevolent Association*, 302 So. 2d, 200, Fla. 1974; *Cidis v. White*, 336 NYS 2d 362, NY, 1972.
10. See, e.g., Holder, Angela: Legal Issues in Pediatrics and Adolescent Medicine, New York, John Wiley, 1977, Chapter VI.
11. 43 *Fed. Reg.* 2084-2114, January 13, 1978.
12. Holder, A: Legal Issues, p 10.
13. 43 *Fed. Reg.* 31786-31794, July 21, 1978.
14. 44 *Fed. Reg.* 24106-24111, April 24, 1979.

1. Eisenberg L: The Social Imperatives of Medical Research. Science, 198: 1105–1110, 1977.
2. Gaylin W, Macklin R: Who Speaks for the Child. The Problems of Proxy Consent. New York, Plenum Press, 1982.
3. Levine RJ: Ethics and Regulation of Clinical Research. Baltimore, Urban & Schwarzenberg, 1981.
4. Melton GB, Koocher GP, Saks MJ: Children's Competence to Consent. Plenum Press, New York, 1983.
5. Walters L: Some Ethical Issues in Research Involving Human Subjects. Ethics Sci Med 6:167, 1979.

SECTION SIX

SOCIETY AND CHILDREN

Physicians have long been involved in caring and working at societal and institutional levels. The medical care of children and adolescents does not occur in a vacuum, but in the midst of complex developing societies. Michael Rothenberg theorizes that there is a national conspiracy against children in the United States. To support his thesis, he presents data in relationship to seven areas in which children function. Next, he proposes an approach to help understand how this state of affairs has come about and makes specific recommendations to remedy this situation. Since it is equally important to highlight well-motivated work on behalf of children, I selected for this anthology the ethical message conveyed by the psychosocial policy guidelines for administration of pediatric health care facilities, as developed by the Association for the Care of Children's Health. The most important issue of our time is the fate of the world, which may be endangered by atomic warfare. Howard Brody contributes for this volume a scholarly essay on this subject, evoking the perspective of the physician who cares for children and their families. To conclude this book dealing with the ethical problems of pediatric practice, Richard Cornelius facilitates the understanding of the legal issues that so often are intertwined with them.

Michael B. Rothenberg, M.D.

17

IS THERE AN UNCONSCIOUS NATIONAL CONSPIRACY AGAINST CHILDREN IN THE UNITED STATES?

This has been a difficult chapter to prepare. The difficulty has been threefold: First of all, I have had to undergo a good deal of frequently painful introspection concerning my own childhood, my feelings about it, and the effect of those feelings on my ability to write this paper; secondly, I have had to engage in a review of my own clinical experiences during nearly twenty-five years as a pediatrician and child psychiatrist working with severely disabled, disturbed, and disadvantaged children and their families, as well as immersing myself in many others' often vividly detailed accounts of their own similar experiences; and finally I have had to struggle to find the balance of factual presentation and personal and professional outrage which, I hope, might move at least some of my readers to action.

In an attempt to set the question posed in my title into a helpful perspective, I want to take at least a brief glimpse into the history of childhood in the Western world. The first attempt at a history of childhood from a psychologic viewpoint was published in 1974 by a group of ten psychohistorians under the leadership of Lloyd DeMause.[1] Their first sentence is, "The history of childhood is a nightmare from which we have only recently begun to awaken." Like the historic biographers, the historic sociologists, and the literary historians, this group of psychohistorians unfolds

Reprinted by courtesy of Clinical Pediatrics 19:10-24, 1980.

a tale of horror, beginning in antiquity, that includes infanticide, abandonment, brutal toilet training, physical discipline which today would universally be called battering, and sexual abuse of every sort and description.

My thesis, in this presentation, is that there is indeed a national conspiracy against children in our country, albeit one that is to a significant degree unconscious for most of the adults participating in it. I present some facts to support my thesis, propose an approach to understanding how this state of affairs has come about, and make some recommendations that I feel will help us move toward a solution to this problem.

SOME FACTS

Americans idealize and romanticize their children more than any other people on the earth. But in the face of this, as Kenneth Keniston has said, "For 200 years Americans have valued the child mainly as a producer—first on the farm, then in the factory and now as a cognitive whiz."

I have limited myself to a very brief survey of data in relation to seven areas in which children function. In these areas, the persistence of negative—if not out-and-out destructive—conditions suggests the presence of a national conspiracy against children.

CHILD ABUSE

At first blush, it appears that there is a great deal of national activity in the area of child abuse. Both professional literature and popular publications abound with articles on the subject. All 50 states have passed child abuse reporting laws. There is even a federal office that concerns itself with this issue. Programs for the prevention and treatment of child abuse have been repeatedly documented as necessary and effective. However, on closer inspection, one discovers that the money and personnel necessary to carry out these programs are simply not available. Indeed, what happened in the State of Washington is not atypical: Within 18 months after passing a mandatory child abuse reporting law, the State Legislature, as part of an overall economy drive, cut the budget for Children's Protective Services in the State by 50%.

The issue of child abuse has, with few exceptions, been dealt with only on one level, that of dealing with the interaction between the abused child and his or her caretaker. David Gil's concept of three levels of child abuse is largely ignored.[2] Gil has attempted to call to our attention the multiple problems of institutional abuse of children (the second level)—in schools, day care settings, correctional institutions, residential treatment centers, and hospitals—about which so little is written or said and even less is being done. Finally, Gil points to a third, and perhaps most important level of abuse—child abuse as a matter of public policy.

Our society's emphasis on conformity is perhaps nowhere more strikingly manifested than in the area of education. When the United States Office of Education asked schools across the country to forward the number of gifted and talented children, more than half responded that there were none—a statistical impossibility. Albert Einstein said,[4]

> It is nothing short of a miracle that the modern methods of instruction have not yet entirely strangled the holy curiosity of inquiry, for this delicate little plant, aside from stimulation, stands mainly in the need of freedom; without this it goes to wrack and ruin without fail. It is a very grave mistake to think that the enjoyment of seeing and searching can be promoted by means of coercion and a sense of duty.

Most recently, we find ourselves confronted with what has been called "the 'elastic mind' movement."[5] Psychologists Bertram Cohler of the University of Chicago, Jerome Kagan of Harvard University, and others are espousing the theory of what Kagan calls "the baby's elastic mind."[6] Their thesis is that the way parents raise their children, and the extent to which the parents themselves might be troubled, doesn't really matter in how the children will turn out, because people keep remaking their lives *all* their lives; and what happens to children later, including what they do for themselves, pretty well compensates for earlier disadvantages and upbringing. This movement ignores the extensive work of such investigators as Klaus and Kennell, Spitz, Broussard, and Fraiberg, to name only a few. Obviously, the "elastic mind" theory could be applied to children in all arenas, not just the educational system.

Let me end this section with Dr. Gilbert Kliman's response to the elastic mind movement:

> We in our culture are finding it increasingly difficult to bear the pain of our children. We no longer have the excuse we used to have when people had large families and could say they were too busy to give each child a lot of individual attention. So we must rationalize our collective neglect of children by denying that the neglect does them any harm. Just as each of us has individually repressed all the painful memories of those earliest, most vulnerable years, we would like to be able to say of children in general: early experience doesn't matter. It all just goes away and is forgotten.[5]

THE LAW AND JUSTICE SYSTEM

With our legacy of English common law, children in the last quarter of the twentieth century in America are still seen as chattels. This idea is dramatically represented by the 1977 United States Supreme Court decision upholding corporal punishment in our public schools: the majority of the Court reasoned that the Eighth Amendment proscribing "cruel and unusual punishment" applies only to criminals and criminal law.

The United States Senate Subcommittee to Investigate Juvenile Delinquency recently reported the following statistics: Although youngsters from 10 to 17 account for only 16% of our population, they account for nearly 50% of all persons arrested for serious crimes; 31% of all crimes solved involved persons younger than 18; the peak age for arrests for violent crime is 18; the peak age for arrests for major property crime is 16.[7]

When the National Commission for Children in Need of Parents met in Seattle at the end of March, 1978, the Captain, who is Commander of the Juvenile Division of the Seattle Police Department, and has himself been a foster parent to 94 abandoned, abused, and neglected children, challenged the Commission to list the constitutional rights of foster children. Pointing out that such rights were listed for parents, Captain Knechtel said, "I'll save you some time. There aren't any. There is no law or statute or anything that lists the rights of foster children." He reminded the Commission that nationally more than 350,000 children live temporarily, sometimes from birth to age 18, in a succession of foster homes, bouncing from foster home to foster home or from their natural parent's home to a foster home and back "like a yo-yo." Knechtel cited research showing that between 60% and 65% of multiple juvenile offenders—those who have had more than five contacts with the police—had their first contact as a neglected, abandoned, or abused child. These multiple juvenile offenders account for 50% of all crime and 70% of all violent crime commited by juveniles.

Howard James' book, *Children in Trouble: A National Scandal,* presents a massive quantity of data in relation to the juvenile justice system.[8] The book is accurately described on its dust jacket as, "A sensitive yet shocking study of the juvenile penal system in America which has consigned more than 300,000 children, some as young as four and five, to the deadening brutality of prisons, reform schools and detention homes."

The Children's Defense Fund of the Washington Research Project has accumulated a great deal of data concerning the inequities of the law and justice system on all levels in this country in relation to children. I would refer those who are interested in more details in this area to their office in Washington, DC.

THE LEGISLATIVE SYSTEM

In December of 1976, Dr. Stephen P. Hersh, Assistant Director for Children and Youth at the National Institute of Mental Health, wrote the following in his Annual Report to the National Advisory Mental Health Council:

There are 106 programs as far as we know relevant to child and maternal health throughout the federal government. These are found within five distinct executive departments. Within these departments the programs are scattered over 15 agencies, 45 offices, bureaus or institutes. . . .These 106 programs expend at least 32 billion dollars a year, of which only 2.2 billion are specifically involved in actual

> health services for children and their mothers. The 106 programs are based on 58 pieces of legislation. These pieces of legislation have passed through almost 30 congressional committees and subcommittees. . . .Coordination, cooperation, similar regulations, similar guidelines, similar standards, similar ways of distributing and allocating of public funds are the exception rather than the rule. We have no National policy. We have no National leadership and commitment at the highest level thus far.

Despite a considerable organizational shake-up at the National Institutes of Health, I can detect no national policy or leadership and commitment at the highest level in the current national administration.

I have said in another context that children have neither money nor the vote and therefore are no politician's constituency.[9] There are, fortunately, some rare exceptions to this view. One of them is ex-Vice President Walter Mondale. While still in the Senate, Vice President Mondale was interviewed by Dr. Milton Senn in connection with Senn's book, *Speaking Out for America's Children.*[3] Among other things, Mondale said, ". . . I don't know of anyone who has studied this field who thinks those programs and their funding or the way in which they are administered in any way approximate the scope of the problem."

The Advisory Committee on Child Development of the National Academy of Science was set up in 1972 to take stock of what was known and to develop recommendations for national policies. They examined the White House Conference Report of 1909 and all the ones since, and concluded that 90% of the recommendations made in 1909 are still suitable today, but that most of these have still not been acted upon in any way by a policy body. As Dr. Orville Brim concluded:[3]

> . . . this implies two things: there is a continuity in what professionals believe is desirable for child-care practices over the past sixty years; and secondly, that the children of the United States do not seem to be an important political constituency. . . .Rather than attempt to hand in another set of items without priorities, we said, "Why not just run off another copy of the 1909 White House Report, put the committee's signature on it, and hand that in?"

THE MASS MEDIA AND CHILDREN

During the past decade, two national commissions and several congressional hearings have addressed themselves to the issue of violence in America generally, and violence on television specifically. A massive amount of documentation now exists which attests to the negative effects of television viewing on children's behavior, on their nutrition, and on their overall psychosocial growth and development. While less is known about the effects of other mass media, such as movies and comic books, there is certainly a strong suggestion that the effects are similarly negative.

Even though these data have been repeatedly presented to appropriate government officials, nothing has been done through either legislative channels or government commissions, such as the Federal Communications Commission, to protect children from this public health hazard which Dr. Anne Somers called, "pollution of the mind."[10] Perhaps this is because 25% of the television industry's profit comes from the 7% of its programming directed at children.

THE ECONOMIC SYSTEM

The Pulitzer Prize-winning investigative reporter, Howard James, in his devastating book, *The Little Victims: How America Treats Its Children*, points out that if there is a State religion in America it is what he would call "hedonistic consumerism."[11] This is an obvious fact of adult life in America to even the most casual observer. What is less apparent is the organized and deliberate manner in which, particularly with the increasingly widespread use of television over the last twenty-five years, the child and adolescent consumer has been targeted by American Industry.

In 2250 BC, the Code of Hammurabi made selling something to a child or buying something from a child without power of attorney a crime punishable by death. In 1978 AD, the average American child will have been exposed to somewhere between 300,000 and 350,000 television commercials alone by the time he reaches age 18. Fifty-five per cent of these commercials are for edibles, 65% of all the food advertised is sugared. Calculating at an average cost of $35,000 per commercial, there is an expenditure of some 700 million dollars annually in television commercials alone.

American children and youth are the targets of multibillion dollar food, clothing, cosmetic, toy, and music industries. The toy industry alone consists of 925 companies which gross a total of 2.8 billion dollars annually.[13] It is shocking to juxtapose this figure with the fact that a government agency has estimated that there are 700,000 toy-related accidents each year in the United States, some 10,000 of them serious enough to lead to the hospitalization of the child.

Perhaps the issues involved in the effect of the economic system on children can best be summarized by the following filler that appeared in the New Yorker Magazine in October, 1977:

"Our Children Are Our Jewels!"
Fashion Lecture

> One of the slides was a woman stepping off a curb holding a little girl by the hand. "Look at this beautiful woman!" said Dorothy Waxman. "Look at the stunning neutral palette of colors she has chosen—the hat just a slightly brighter shade than the jacket. The colors aren't flashy, but they really come alive. And look at the beautiful blonde little girl. What a wonderful accessory!"

Unconscious Conspiracy?

In January 1978, a panel of medical experts was called together by Representative James H. Scheuer (D.—NY) for two days of hearings on possible revisions to the US Maternal and Child Health Act, under consideration in Congress.

Representative Scheuer cited the following figures:

- Some 10 million children younger than age 16 receive no medical care whatever in this country.
- About half of all children in the United States less than the age of 15 have never seen a dentist.
- 19 million children are not fully immunized against polio.
- 14 million children are unprotected against measles and German measles.

At the same hearings, Dr. Saul Robinson, President of the American Academy of Pediatrics, pointed out that between 1960 and 1975, federal health dollars invested in child health declined from one of every two to one of every ten spent. Dr. Robinson said, "The early formative years require better health service, yet we still have not adopted a national policy for promoting health, preventing disease and illness, and guaranteeing our youngest citizens the right to a healthy future."

It has been estimated that at least 10 million of the 67 million school children in the country need help for psychologic disturbances if they are to complete successfully their school work. There are over 2 million severely disturbed adolescents housed in state hospitals and correctional institutions. Despite these figures, and the fact that there are fewer than 2500 trained child psychiatrists in the country, with other child mental health professionals in equally short supply, the training of all child mental health workers has been sharply curtailed in recent years.

Although they make up 40% of the population, children and adolescents receive less than 5% of available mental health services in the country.

The concept of therapeutic play, particularly as a way to prevent emotional trauma in an enormous variety of hospital situations, remains unknown to most physicians and nurses and poorly understood by the vast majority of those who are even aware of it. No more than a handful of all children's hospitals in the country have child life and education programs which are funded out of the basic, annual hospital budget. Restriction of visiting hours remains the rule in most children's medical settings, particularly in relation to visits from young siblings. It is my conviction that children's hospitals are still run for the convenience of the adults who work in them, with only a secondary focus on the needs of the children treated in them.

If it feels as if I have burdened the reader with too many awesome and awful statistics, I can only say these represent a very small proportion of the mass I have accumulated during the past few years.

How did this "conspiracy" against children begin, and how is it sustained at the present time?

DeMause postulates that when an adult is face to face with a child who needs something, the adult has three major reactions available: (1) He can use the child as a vehicle for projecting the contents of his own unconscious (projective reaction); (2) he can use the child as a substitute for an adult figure important in his own childhood (reversal reaction); or, (3) he can empathize with the child's needs and act to satisfy them (empathic reaction).[1] While the projective and reversal reactions are far more common in the past history of childhood, they remain all too familiar today, as in the common reversal reaction of the child batterer who says, "When he cried, it meant he didn't love me. So I hit him."

In a Commentary in *Pediatrics* in the fall of 1977 I said:[13]

> A lot of people go into pediatrics because they are more comfortable with children than they are with adults or because they have an urgent need to be in total control of their patients—or even out of classical reaction formation, *i.e.*, reacting against their basic dislike of and discomfort with children by doing exactly the opposite of their impulse and spending most of their time working with children. Individuals who have chosen pediatrics for any of these reasons are obviously not going to be interested in becoming very involved in psychosocial and behavioral issues, since such involvement would inevitably lead to their being confronted with their own motivations for going into the field. I think we need to bring this hidden agenda out in the open and build in answers to the questions it raises, within our pediatric training program . . ."

While I am far less familiar with others who work with children than I am with pediatricians and child psychiatrists, I feel that similar processes often underlie the decision of people to enter other professions and vocations that primarily involve work with children.

It is my impression, then, that the "national conspiracy" against children has been produced by and is sustained by these projective reactions, reversal reactions, and reaction formations which are largely unconscious in all of us, or of which we are only superficially and transiently aware.

I feel that very few of us are fortunate enough to enter adulthood without a frightened, hurt, and angry child still very much alive within us. It seems to me that this is what causes each of us to suppress or repress an awareness of these projective and reversal reactions and reaction formations—unless we make a major, conscious effort to bring our feelings out into the open and work them through.

RECOMMENDATIONS

I would urge those interested in becoming involved in a broad-based child advocacy plan on a community level to spend five minutes familiarizing themselves with Howard James' Lafayette Plan. James' plan was developed in Lafayette, Indiana in May 1971, and in time became the basis of a statewide advocacy group for children.[11] The details are laid out in seven pages in his book. Suffice it to say that with minimal guidance from James, two women in the community with less than $1000 in start-up money were able to launch a full-scale advocacy program for children and youth.

For those of us who spend our working lives in the child health care field, I am calling for a national campaign, to be supported by a consortium of all the organizations to which we belong. The campaign will have three objectives: First, to get in touch with our ambivalence about children and youth to the point that we can—second, take a leadership role in helping all others who work with children to a similar awareness of their ambivalence so that—third, we may all be able to work together, *focused on the needs of children,* rather than on the power, "turf," and money issues which have so fragmented and effectively destroyed our efforts to bring about substantive changes for the children of America.

I know that it's an awesome task to confront one's ambivalence about children. But I'm convinced that we can go about it in a practical way which doesn't involve each of us in long-term psychotherapy.

The first step is for each one to accept that it's at least possible that he or she has negative feelings toward children.

Second, one must ask oneself what it is that one really wants from one's work with children and adolescents.

Third, we have to recognize that it's easier for us in the health care field to be care*givers* than care*takers*. That is, we *give* care *to* others easily, but it's much harder for us to *take* care *from* others. This is important, because each of us will have to turn to coworkers and colleagues for support, while we undergo the painful process of getting in touch with the angry and resentful feelings which we experience during our work with children and their families. This is formally called peer group support and consultation.

Fourth, we may have to engage in small group workshops and seminars (*not* "encounter" or "sensitivity" groups) with consultants from *outside* the group who have special skills in helping working groups engage in mutually-supportive self-examination.

Fifth, we shall have to work together to convince administrators in our work settings that the time and money needed for this process is not a luxury, but a critical necessity for the provision of quality services to children and their families.

A FINAL WORD

For those who work in health care settings for children, let me suggest the prayer of Sir Robert Hutchison, a 19th Century English pediatrician, as a guide to meeting human needs in the context of political realities:

From inability to let well alone;
from too much zeal for the new
and contempt for what is old;
from putting knowledge before wisdom,
science before art, and cleverness before
common sense;
from treating patients as cases, and from
making the cure of the disease more
grievous than the endurance of the same,
Good Lord, deliver us.

REFERENCES

1. DeMause L (ed): The History of Childhood. New York, The Psychohistory Press, a Division of ATCON, Inc. Publishers, 1974, p 1.
2. Gil DG: Violence against Children: Physical Child Abuse in the US. Cambridge, Harvard University Press, 1970, pp 1–204.
3. Senn MJE: Speaking Out for America's Children. London, Yale University Press. 1977, section 1, p 3.
4. Aring CD: Creativity requires nurture (commentary). JAMA 237:1205, 1977.
5. Rosenfeld A: The elastic mind movement: rationalizing child neglect? Saturday Rev, Apr 1, 1978, pp 26–28.
6. Kagan J: The baby's elastic mind. Human Nature 1:1, 1978.
7. Juvenile Crime. Article in Seattle Post-Intelligencer Parade Magazine, July 11, 1976.
8. James H: Children in Trouble: A National Scandal. New York. David McKay Company Inc. 1970, pp 1–287; pocket book edition, 1971.
9. Rothenberg MB: The effect of television violence on children and youth. JAMA 234:1043, 1975.
10. Somers AR: Violence, television and the health of American youth. N Engl J Med 294:811, 1976.
11. James H: The Little Victims: How America Treats Its Children. New York, David McKay Company Inc, 1975, p 1–374.
12. Kent A: Chairman of the Board, Toy Manufacturers Association, in testimony to the Children and Advertising Seminar Series of the Georgetown University Law Center, April 19, 1977.
13. Rothenberg MB: Child psychiatry and pediatrics. Commentary on child psychiatry and pediatrics: The state of the relationship. Anders TF. Pediatrics 60:649, 1977.

Lynn Gordon
Susan Kleinberg
Mary E. McCarthy
Constance U. Battle

18

PSYCHOSOCIAL POLICY GUIDELINES FOR ADMINISTRATION OF PEDIATRIC HEALTH CARE FACILITIES

I. EQUALITY AND RESPECT

A. EQUAL TREATMENT

What The Health Care Setting Must Do

The health care setting should ensure that each child and family is treated equally, with dignity and respect, and with an appreciation for the family's life-style, customs, language, culture, and diet. Regardless of the type of facility (whether or not it is specifically a pediatric hospital, general hospital with a pediatric department or hospital with no pediatric department), each child should have every opportunity for care that is appropriate to his/her age group, including staff trained to work with children.

Explanation

Without exception, all children are entitled to the best available care regardless of their own or their family's race, color, language, physical or

Reprinted with permission of the Association for the Care of Children's Health.

mental status, religion, national origin, political opinion, socioeconomic status, or sex.

Specific Recommendations

The health care setting should:

1. instruct all staff that respectful treatment is to be accorded each child and family.
2. assign children to appropriate units within the hospital so that adequate care for the child's particular age group and diagnosis can be provided. Children of similar ages and abilities should be grouped together. At no time should a child share a room with an adult.
3. provide a translator when there is a language barrier.
4. provide a diet which is in keeping with the customs of the family, insofar as this is possible.

B. CONFIDENTIALITY

What The Health Care Setting Must Do

The health care setting should provide for the child's (and his/her family's) right to confidentiality throughout the entire care process and afterwards.

Explanation

The child and the family need to know that they are protected from embarrassment and distress which could be caused by public knowledge of their intimate personal affairs. Only when they feel that their privacy is guarded will they feel free to cooperate fully and honestly in the course of treatment.

Each member of the health care team must preserve confidentiality in all matters, both in the keeping of medical records, and in discussions regarding the child, his/her family, history, diagnosis, and treatment. This policy must apply in all situations, including the provisions of birth control services, treatment for venereal diseases, care relating to conditions of pregnancy, seeking and obtaining of psychiatric care and counseling, and care for substance abuse (drugs, alcohol, etc.).

Specific Recommendations

The health care setting should:

1. limit access to a child's records to authorized personnel only.

2. limit discussions regarding patient care and treatment to those persons who need to be informed.
3. when appropriate, code medical charges confidentially for billing purposes.

C. ACKNOWLEDGMENT OF THE CHILD

What The Health Care Setting Must Do

The health care setting should ensure that by their language and behavior all members of the staff acknowledge the child as a person, not as an inanimate object, not as a disease or condition. The individuality of each child must be respected.

Explanation

All children are entitled to the full dignity and respect they deserve by virtue of their humanity and intrinsic personal worth. Their treatment in any setting should reflect a true concern for their physical and emotional comfort.

Specific Recommendations

The health care setting should:

1. instruct all staff to treat the child with courtesy, including greeting the child by name, introducing unfamiliar staff, and talking to the child directly rather than using the third person.
2. ensure that the child is either included in any discussion (consultation, rounds, etc.) or that the discussion is delayed until a time when the child is not present.

D. ROUNDS AT THE CHILD'S BEDSIDE

What The Health Care Setting Must Do

The health care setting should ensure that medical and other personnel will limit their discussion in the presence of the child to conversation that is beneficial and instructive for the child, and that is geared to his/her cognitive, emotional, social, and language development.

Explanation

Rounds at the bedside must not include discussion for the education of medical and/or other personnel unless it is thoroughly appropriate that the child hear the proceedings. Too frequently, the child is treated as an object or disease with no thoughts and feelings of his/her own. The child is left no recourse but to imagine or fantasize about the meaning of the conversation at his/her own developmental level. This can result in frightening misperceptions about a child's condition and treatment.

Specific Recommendations

The health care setting should:

1. instruct all staff that conversation occurring at the child's bedside, or anywhere within the child's hearing, be directed to the child and geared to his/her level of comprehension. All such discussion should be appropriate for the child to hear.
2. ensure that discussion or conversation that must occur among professionals will take place out of the child's hearing.
3. provide follow-up conversation with a child who demonstrates a misunderstanding of his/her condition or treatment.

E. PROTECTION OF PRIVACY

What The Health Care Setting Must Do

The health care setting should ensure that the privacy and delicate feelings of each child about his/her body are protected at all times.

Explanation

Every child is a human being and has the right to be treated with dignity and respect, as well as the right to refuse being put on display and potentially embarrassed in front of others regardless of the rationalizations of the medical personnel. Most children will not be able to refuse invasions of their privacy.

Specific Recommendations

The health care setting should:

1. make sure that no staff member will conduct treatments, procedures, or physical examinations in playrooms, hallways, or other public places.
2. provide treatment rooms accessible to the child's unit.
3. make sure that curtains or screens are placed around a child's bed when a treatment, procedure, or physical examination is conducted in multiple-bed rooms.

F. INFORMING THE CHILD

What The Health Care Setting Must Do

The health care setting should provide adequate and appropriate explanations to the child so that he/she fully understands the reasons for and specific details regarding the health care to be provided.

Explanation

In order to cope with illness, medical procedures, and hospitalization in general, a child needs to know what is being done to him/her now and what treatment plans for the future include. This approach will limit misunderstandings, fears, and fantasies which might seriously impede recovery or cause secondary emotional or psychologic trauma.

Specific Recommendations

The health care setting should:

1. instruct the interdisciplinary team to inform the child in simple, developmentally appropriate language why he/she is in the health care facility and what the treatment will entail.
2. assign a team member to ascertain that the child has correctly understood the explanation that he/she has been given.
3. encourage the child to express his/her perceptions and fantasies.
4. instruct a team member to correct a child's misperceptions if necessary.

II. FAMILY INVOLVEMENT

A. MAINTAINING FAMILY TIES

What The Health Care Setting Must Do

The health care setting should provide the opportunity for families to maintain close and continuous relationships when a child requires hospitalization.

Explanation

Separation and illness create anxiety and stress for children. Young children may feel abandoned by their parents, and may view the separation as permanent. This stress can be minimized by encouraging the presence of family members in order to provide emotional support and approximate familiar patterns and routines of care. Parents, however, may be stressed or overemotional when their child is hospitalized. Memories of their own hospitalization as children and other separation experiences may make them incapable of providing emotional care or even routine physical care for their child. Staffing patterns should be adequate to provide appropriate patient care whether the parents are present or not. Thus the hospital must not view a child's parents as ancilliary staff.

Specific Recommendations

The health care setting should:

1. recognize the primary role of the parents as caregivers, and make formal arrangements that allow them to assume as much or as little care for the child as they feel comfortable with, and as is consonant with sound medical practice.
2. post visiting hours, indicating that parents are allowed to visit around-the-clock.
3. encourage parents to remain with the child as much as possible, and provide rooming-in facilities whenever feasible. Where rooming-in is not possible, be flexible in providing some other temporary sleeping arrangement within the hospital.
4. plan hospital stays for children to be as short as possible. In order to avoid undue separation, outpatient procedures should be the first choice whenever possible.
5. set specific policies to facilitate sibling visiting privileges.
6. ensure the free exchange of information: (a) from family to staff, regarding the child's usual behavior patterns and coping mechanisms; and (b) from staff to family, regarding the child's condition and adaptation to the condition and/or health care setting.
7. obtain information about family cultural, religious, or personal routines, and be flexible in accommodating these differences whenever possible.
8. provide written information for distribution to parents covering all hospital policies and procedures pertaining to children (ie, accompanying a child to a procedure, rights of patients and parents).

B. SUPPORTING AND PREPARING FAMILIES

What The Health Care Setting Must Do

The health care setting should provide support and preparation for parents which will enable them, in turn, to support their child.

Explanation

The confusion and anxiety of parents in stressful situations is often transmitted to the child, increasing his/her own anxiety. Support for and preparation of parents can aid them in providing emotional strength for the child.

Specific Recommendations

The health care setting should:

1. explain all procedures to parents, and allow them the privacy and time to assimilate medical information.
2. reinforce oral explanations with printed teaching materials.
3. offer counseling to parents, which allows them time to work through their own feelings.
4. offer parent support groups to help families cope with stress of illness and hospitalization.

III. PREPARATION OF THE CHILD AND FAMILY FOR THE HEALTH CARE EXPERIENCE

A. ROUTINE EDUCATION OF FAMILIES IN THE COMMUNITY

What The Health Care Setting Must Do

The health care setting should ensure that children and families in the community are given varied opportunities to learn about health care facilities and practices before there is any indication that they will need to use them.

Explanation

A child who is sick or hurt is less likely to cope well with the unfamiliar environment and potentially painful experiences of hospitalization or clinic visits. Similarly, the families of such children tend to be anxious and upset. It is important that as many children and families as possible have advance knowledge of what various health care settings are like, and what occurs routinely during a hospital admission or clinic visit.

Specific Recommendations

The health care setting should:

1. develop out-reach programs which include visits to preschools, kindergartens, and other child groups to present interesting and relatively nonthreatening aspects of hospitals and health care.
2. initiate tours of school groups, during which children and adolescents can visit the health care facility and become familiar with the sights, smells, and sounds that they encounter there. Tours might be incorporated into a class curriculum or theme such as 'Community Helpers' or 'Careers.'
3. send staff to participate in the meetings of PTAs and other parent groups, explaining common childhood and adolescent health problems, typical reactions of children to those problems, and the importance of attention to the psychosocial and emotional aspects of health care for children.

B. ADEQUATE EXPLANATION

What The Health Care Setting Must Do

The health care setting should ensure the children and their parents are informed, understand, and have the opportunity to review and discuss experiences of separation, diagnosis, and treatment. These experiences are potentially stressful to any and all members of the family.

Explanation

A child needs to be protected from overwhelming anxiety resulting from fear of the unknown. A child obtains some sense of control from knowing what is to come and having sufficient time to prepare for it. This need for adequate preparation is especially important for any child who is handicapped in his/her capacity to understand, by virtue of serious illness or emotional, cognitive, or social deprivation. It is equally important for young children (less than five years of age) because of their fragmentary understanding of the concepts of time, health, and illness.

Specific Recommendations

The health care setting should:

1. provide the child with an opportunity for a preadmission visit to: (a) meet the staff; (b) become familiar with the hospital environment; (c) have the opportunity to ask questions and discuss what he/she has seen.
2. instruct staff to meet the child and family and provide such a tour soon after admission, if a preadmission tour is not possible.
3. direct staff to ensure that the child and family learn the names of

those who are responsible for his/her direct care, in particular, which physician is responsible for the care. For the child who can read, his/her family, and all hospital staff and volunteers, a card should be taped to the bedstand with the first and last names of the child's hospital caretakers.

4. provide an explanation of communication channels as soon as possible after admission.
5. develop a routine procedure for informing a child and his/her parents concerning the diagnosis, prognosis, and treatment, in language which is readily understandable.
6. make specific provisions for special circumstances in which impediments to communication exist (ie, limited understanding of child or family, language barriers, hearing impairment, chaotic or unstable family).
7. provide a specific opportunity each day for the child and family to ask pertinent questions concerning the diagnosis and treatment, tests, and procedures performed.

C. ACCEPTANCE

What The Health Care Setting Must Do

The health care setting should ensure that children and their families are given the time and assistance they require to come to an appropriate acceptance of the diagnosis, prognosis, treatment, and sequelae associated with the condition of disease which they face.

Explanation

Manageable anticipatory anxiety facilitates a more complete working through of thoughts and feelings, which ultimately leads to a better acceptance of the procedure or consequences. In any life change, such as loss or diminution of function, a mourning or grieving process must take place. A child needs sufficient time and assistance for this process. He/she deserves the developmental challenge of facing a new experience, of learning about it, and of adjusting to it. Parents may need additional support and possibly formal counseling during this process.

Specific Recommendations

1. Provide each child with an appropriate length of time to prepare himself/herself for any particular procedure to the fullest extent that it is medically feasible and in accordance with the child's developmental age and individual coping skills. A sufficient period should be allowed as well for a child to work through life changes that will result

either from the disease or condition itself or from the treatment.

2. Develop a staff structure and pattern which gives serious attention to providing: (a) basic, general emotional support from all hospital staff; (b) indirect intervention by helping the parents support the child; (c) explanations, guidance, and instruction in practical techniques of coping with specific life changes on a day-to-day basis from nurses or the appropriate therapist; (d) direct intervention by a mental health professional, using play therapy, art, and literature, or, for older children, the more conventional types of therapy.

IV. PARTICIPATION BY THE CHILD AND FAMILY IN DISCUSSION AND DECISION-MAKING

What The Health Care Setting Must Do

The health care setting should ensure that the child and his/her parents have opportunities to participate in decision-making, in collaboration with health care professionals.

Explanation

A child has the need to participate in the discussion and consideration of medical or surgical treatment, and to consider the refusal to consent in those instances where the prognosis is clearly poor, and/or the treatments would interfere with other objectives more important to the child and family, such as 'peaceful final days.' Every child has the right to have his/her wishes and preferences given serious consideration when decisions are being made regarding course of treatment, including discontinuation of treatment for a terminally ill child. A child's sense of self-determination and feelings of control are enhanced when he/she has input into the decision-making process. Not only does this participation serve the practical purpose of increasing the child's cooperation, and possibly putting him/her into a frame of mind where maximum benefits from treatment can occur, but it is in accord with a general policy of respecting the right of any person to have a say (for adults, 'informed consent') in what will happen in his/her life.

Specific Recommendations

The health care setting should:

1. encourage staff to develop a written philosophy of patient and parent participation which acknowledges their right to participate as well as the beneficial outcome of such mutual collaboration.
2. assess the extent to which a child can participate in planning for

his/her health care based upon the child's age, emotional maturity, and most of all, on the cognitive ability to perceive and understand clearly the following: (a) alternatives; (b) chance which the therapy has of being successful; (c) degree to which it is thought that the child will be returned to normal or near normal functioning; and (d) potential pain, discomfort, or traumatic side effects.

3. develop a comprehensive interdisciplinary discharge plan which takes into account family needs and preferences.

V. ENVIRONMENT AND DAILY STRUCTURE

A. PROVISION OF DEVELOPMENTALLY APPROPRIATE OPPORTUNITIES

What The Health Setting Must Do

The health care setting should provide every child with the opportunity to participate in developmentally appropriate educational, recreational, and social activities, such as those offered by child life specialists and hospital teachers.

Explanation

Children in hospitals and outpatient clinics need to have their emotional, social, educational, and recreational needs addressed in order to maintain normal routines, facilitate development, and alleviate anxiety and stress. Child life programs, staffed by skilled, sensitive child care professionals, are an essential component of health care because they provide children, through play, with the chance to impose control and demonstrate mastery in at least one aspect of their lives. Educational programs that cater to individual needs are also extremely important to help hospitalized children maintain and improve their academic skills, so as not to fall behind in their regular school work.

Specific Recommendations

The health care setting should:

1. provide professional child life specialists in ratios sufficient to ensure adequate developmental programming and emotional support.
2. provide the services of licensed teachers (either directly through hospital employment, or by an arrangement with the local school system) who will continue a child's education, helping him or her to maintain and improve important academic skills, so as not to fall far behind in regular school work.

3. appoint a child/family advocate, either a nurse or physician, to oversee the quality of care of children in hospitals which have no specific designated pediatric beds.
4. set aside adequate space for activities, separate from other areas, and appropriately designed for the population served.
5. allot an appropriate budget to provide suitable educational and recreational materials and equipment.
6. train all staff and volunteers in an ongoing fashion to ensure their continuing educational development. Child life specialists should offer consultation to other departments so that emotional care will be consistent and continuous.

B. PROVISION OF "SAFE" TIMES

What The Health Care Setting Must Do

The health care setting should provide specific "safe" times for each child on a daily basis, time which will be free of any unexpected or painful experiences.

Explanation

Children in hospitals are required to undergo treatments and therapy that are often painful and/or frightening. These are usually scheduled to meet the varying needs of staff, and often result in the inability of the child to control any aspect of his/her schedule or environment. Specific free time, scheduled daily, allows a child some control, and the freedom from fear of unexpected pain.

Specific Recommendations

The health care setting should:

1. schedule a time each day to allow a child some "safe" time. This should be noted on the nursing care plan, and respected by all staff.
2. instruct staff that painful treatment not be given to the child without warning and explanation, and should never be given in playrooms, lounges, or other public areas.

C. APPROPRIATE PHYSICAL ENVIRONMENT

What The Health Care Setting Must Do

The health care setting should provide an environment for every child which is planned and scaled to his/her needs and reflects the child's individuality.

Explanation

Every child has the right to surroundings in which it is both safe and functional for him/her to move around independently. It is important for the child's development and maintenance of self-esteem that he/she be given as much independence in functioning as possible. The individual identity of each child is important and must be supported.

Specific Recommendations

The health care setting should:

1. provide bathroom facilities, beds, tables, chairs, and doorknobs that are built in such a way that children can use them independently, without an adult's assistance.
2. if necessary, design, construct, or remodel all furniture and equipment so that it will be at the appropriate height for reach or grasp by a child.
3. encourage display of child's personal belongings or artwork.

D. ALLOWING THE CHILD TO TAKE CARE OF HIS/HER OWN NEEDS

What The Health Care Setting Must Do

The health care setting should encourage the child to engage in his/her own daily care activities to the fullest extent possible, including bathing, feeding, toileting, dressing, and ambulating.

Explanation

When the child is allowed to take care of his/her own needs as far as possible, he/she will be better able to maintain self-esteem through continued control over those functions that have been mastered prior to hospitalization.

Specific Recommendations

The health care setting should:

1. instruct all staff to allow adequate time each day so that the child is able to bathe, feed, and dress himself/herself as far as possible.
2. ensure that staff encourages the child to continue using the daily care skills that he/she had achieved prior to hospitalization.
3. permit children to wear their own night clothes or play clothes when possible.

What The Health Care Setting Must Do

The health care setting should ensure that each child is seen promptly. In addition, the facility staff should attend to the whole child, and not limit its attention to the ostensible reason for admission to that facility.

Explanation

A child needs to be attended to within a reasonable time-frame. His/her limited ability to comprehend concepts of time during periods of heightened anxiety or uneasiness makes prompt health care attention an essential component of any care delivery system.

A child has the need for his/her special needs to be identified as soon as possible in order to prevent future disability and maximize the benefits of health care intervention and to make true comprehensive health care available to him/her. All children, insofar as possible, have the right to early detection of any abnormality or deviation in infancy (or as early as possible). They also have the right to immediate and continuing health guidance and comprehensive service until the maximum potential of the child is achieved.

Specific Recommendations

The health care setting should:

1. schedule appointments on a realistic basis.
2. assign staff so that periods of heavy usage are adequately covered.
3. encourage staff to explain when the system fails.
4. when appropriate, provide play opportunities for the child.
5. ensure that the child, a constantly changing individual, is evaluated by a multidisciplinary team at reasonable intervals.
6. ensure that suspicions about delays or gaps in cognitive, social, motor, and sensory development are pursued.
7. instruct each staff member to treat the whole child, and to review and discuss the child with other professionals through multidisciplinary meetings.

SUGGESTED READINGS

Adams MA: A hospital play program: helping children with serious illness. Am J Orthopsychiatry 3:46, 1976.

Belmont HS: Hospitalization and its effect upon the total child. Clin Pediatr 9, 1970.

Freud A: The role of bodily illness in the mental life of children. Psychoanalytic Study of the Child 7:69, 1952.

Gellert E (ed): Psychosocial aspects of pediatric care. New York, Grune & Stratton, 1978.

Glaser H: The hospital as an environment. J Assoc Care of Children in Hosp 1:3, 1974.

Haggerty R, Klaus J, Roghmann J, Pless IB: Child health and the community. New York, Wiley-Interscience, 1975.

Klaus M, Kennell J: Maternal infant-bonding. St. Louis, C.V. Mosby, 1976.

Lawson BA: Chronic illness in the school-age child: Effects on the total family. Maternal Child Nursing, January-February, 1977.

Murphy LB: The widening world of childhood: Paths toward mastery. New York, Basic Books, Inc., 1962.

Petrillo M, Sanger S: Emotional care of hospitalized children, 2nd ed. Philadelphia, J.B. Lippincott, 1980.

Plank E: Working with children in hospitals. Chicago, Year Book Medical Publishers, 1971.

Prugh D, et al: A study of the emotional reactions of children and their families to hospitalization. Am J Orthopsychiatry 70, 1953.

Robertson J: Young child in hospital. London, Tavistock Publications, 1970.

Robinson ME: Psychological impact of illness and hospitalization on the child: birth through 12 years. Paper presented at a meeting of the Metropolitan-Washington affiliate of ACCH, May, 1972.

Rothenberg M: Is there a national conspiracy against children in the United States? *In* Human Needs and Political Realities. Washington, DC, US Government Printing Office, 1978.

Shore M: Red is the color of hurting. Washington DC, US Government Printing Office, 1965.

Skipper JK, Leonard RC: Children, stress, and hospitalization: A field experiment. J Health Soc Behav 9, 1965.

Spitz R: Hospitalism: An inquiry into the genesis of psychiatric conditions in early childhood. Psychoanalytic Study of the Child 43, 1945.

Starfield B, Barkowe S: Physician recognition of complaints made by parents about their children's health. Pediatrics 43, 1969.

Study to quantify the uniqueness of children's hospitals. Wilmington, Del: National Association of Children's Hospitals and Related Institutions, 1978.

Tisza V, Angoff K: A play program and its function in a pediatric hospital. Pediatrics 19, 1957.

Vardaro JA: Pre-admission anxiety and mother-child relationships. J Assoc Care of Child in Hosp 2:7, 1978.

Wolfer JA Visintainer M: Pediatric surgical patients' stress responses and adjustments. Nursing Research 24, 1975.

Howard Brody, M.D., Ph.D.

19

NUCLEAR ARMS AND THE SOCIAL RESPONSIBILITY OF THE PEDIATRICIAN

INTRODUCTION

While the nuclear arms race and the threat of nuclear war are most commonly viewed as political problems, they are also moral issues in the most profound sense. Since there is reasonable scientific evidence to suggest that a widespread nuclear war would threaten the existence of the human race on this planet, the possible consequences of nuclear war include a moral outrage compared with which even genocide is a relative peccadillo. Furthermore, it may be argued that the threat of nuclear annihilation casts a pall over the moral climate of our contemporary society. As Jonathan Schell has depicted in dramatic terms, our present culture is perched at the edge of a nuclear abyss, fearing to push the button and tumble over the edge, but fearing equally to take definitive action to rebuild itself at a safer location far back from the brink.[1] At one level, members of this society are vaguely aware of their schizophrenic role as their own potential executioners and simultaneously their own potential victims. Yet at another level the life of society goes on as before, as everyone participates in a massive denial of this abyss and of their mutual conscious decision to choose to live on the edge of it. Such a culture does not seem to be one well situated for adherence to deeply ingrained moral values, or for engaging in thoughtful moral reflection of its plight. If one wonders at the moral decay and moral chaos exhibited by this culture, one perhaps need look no farther than the imminent threat of nuclear destruction for the cause of this dismal state of affairs.

Anyone concerned about the future of the human race and the health and longevity of its members ought to feel a profound urge to grapple with this moral dilemma, arguably the most important moral issue facing our society today. This should be especially true of anyone whose primary interest is the growth and development of children and adolescents. Later in this chapter, I offer an argument, based in large part on an analogy to other obligations and issues of public health, to support the physician's responsibility in the prevention of nuclear war. I also suggest some reasons why practitioners of pediatrics and adolescent medicine might feel a special responsibility in this regard.

Before turning to these substantive arguments, however, I would like to address directly some possible objections to my approach. I do this at the outset of the chapter for two reasons. First, it is likely that the reader who holds these objections, and who has heard no effective reply to them, will tend to resist being persuaded by any arguments I might offer. Second, some of what I say in reply to these objections has general applicability to medical ethics generally, and may be of interest totally apart from the nuclear issue. The objections I wish to address are the following three:

1. The argument for the physician's social responsibility in the nuclear war issue is casuistic. Certain physicians, for reasons that grow out of their own personal political philosophies, have chosen to take strong antinuclear stances. They then try to browbeat their fellow physicians into joining them by framing apparently logical arguments in their support. However, the conclusion of these arguments is known in advance, and so the arguments themselves amount to narrow partisanship rather than open-minded moral reflection.

2. The magnitude of the horrors of nuclear war, ranging from the sheer numbers of dead and injured on the macro level to the individual vignettes of suffering and terror among the survivors of Hiroshima and Nagasaki on the micro level, lend themselves to a rhetoric overkill that eliminates the possibility for a rational discussion of the issues. In this regard, the medical opponents of nuclear war (members of organizations like the Physicians for Social Responsibility and the International Physicians for the Prevention of Nuclear War) are no different from those antiabortion supporters who believe that they can persuade the rest of the public to join their cause by showing gory pictures of aborted fetuses.

3. While it is all very well to pretend that discussion of the terrors of nuclear war is an exercise in continuing physician education or a discussion of medical morality, inevitably any such conversation soon wanders into the realm of politics. At this point, legitimate medical expertise ends, and physicians are being asked to take a stand on territory that is foreign to them as professionals.

Since the first two of these three objections are closely related, I next turn to a brief discussion of the role of casuistry and rhetoric in medical ethics, in the hopes of showing that these terms, usually used with negative connotation only, in fact have a positive side which is relevant to the issues at hand.

CASUISTRY AND RHETORIC IN MEDICAL ETHICS

Discussion of the pediatrician's moral responsibility for the prevention of nuclear war may include elements of casuistry and rhetoric. In contemporary usage, these terms are used almost exclusively in a derogatory sense. We are indebted to one of the more thoughtful scholars in medical ethics, Albert Jonsen, for reminding us that casuistry and rhetoric are both intellectual disciplines with a long and distinguished history and with their own rigorous methodologies; indeed some methodologic problems in modern medical ethics might be resolved if we were to rediscover our roots in those intellectual disciplines.[2] It is in this scholarly sense about which Jonsen has reminded us, rather than in the usual derogatory sense, that I propose to use these terms.

The casuists were a school of Medieval and early Renaissance scholars whose method of case-study analysis eventually deteriorated to the point where their critics felt that they would use legalistic rationalization to justify any course of action proposed—hence the disrepute into which the term has fallen. Applied properly, however, casuistry should be no stranger to anyone who has tried to analyze issues in medical ethics with a case-study approach. The best casuists first selected cases that seemed to illustrate moral rules or principles in the clearest possible way. Around each paradigm case they then assembled a cluster of related cases, arranged in an orderly sequence so that one went by gradual degrees from those cases most closely resembling the paradigm case in all morally relevant respects, through those cases that differed from the paradigm case in some respects but not in others, until one reached the fringe cases where the applicability of the moral rule was most tenuous. For each case the proper degree and scope of the applicability of the moral rule was discussed, with a lively awareness of the real-life circumstances embodied in the case description. The casuist tried to argue rationally which sorts of circumstances were fully consistent with the moral rule; which required some modification of the rule (or produced overlap with a different and conflicting moral rule); and which changed the nature of the case so much that the rule no longer applied. Finally, the casuist appended to each case analysis some label reflecting the degree of certainty represented by the conclusion—which case analyses were felt to be thoroughly defensible and which were felt to be more tenuous owing to gaps in the supporting arguments. Jonsen, in reviewing this scholarly method, concludes that contemporary work in medical ethics fits this "good" casuistry model better than it does the various "applied ethics" models that many have proposed.

Casuistic sorts of arguments appear frequently in the debate over nuclear weapons, as they do in other medical-ethical issues. For example, one of the best analyses to date, by Cassel and Jameton, relies heavily on the analogy between the physician's taking responsibility to oppose the nuclear arms race and the physician who, in nineteenth century London, defied the law and the utility companies to remove the handle from a public pump, thereby calling attention to a contaminated water source that was spreading cholera.[3] A full discussion would require careful analysis of the points of analogy and dysanalogy between the public-health, preventive-medicine paradigm case and the nuclear-war case (degree of physician expertise, ability of individual physicians to effect change, and so forth).

The term "rhetoric" is now generally used to refer to an argument that could not succeed on its own merits, but persuades the listener only by use of flowery phrases, double-talk, or some other superficial trickery. It is thus easy for us to forget that rhetoric was also a well-respected intellectual discipline, in fact one of the seven central fields of study in the original universities. Scholars of the Aristotelian tradition distinguished carefully between different fields of human inquiry, arguing that depending on the subject matter, different degrees of certainty could be achieved. Mathematics was the extreme case of a field in which a high degree of certainty was attainable; and those sciences like astronomy to which mathematics could be readily applied could thereby expect a similarly high level of certainty. In many fields having to do with practical human affairs, however, certainty of this sort was simply unobtainable, and even the most careful inquiry and study could reveal answers that were not *certain* but only *highly probable*. To reject a probable explanation in such fields just because it falls short of mathematical certainty indicates not commendable intellectual rigor, but instead a misunderstanding of the degree of certainty that the field will allow. The goal of rhetoric, then, was to provide rational arguments within those fields of inquiry for which certainty was unobtainable. Since practical human affairs require action, a goal of rhetoric was to present rational argument in a way that appeals to the emotions of the listener, and thus enjoins to positive action rather than appearing merely as a sterile intellectual exercise. The emotional appeal should, however, flow naturally from the reasonableness of the arguments, and cannot be a substitute for reasonableness.

What follows in this dicussion is, I hope, an exercise in rhetoric in the positive sense. Those who agree with my perspectives on nuclear weapons should find thier positions strengthened, perhaps with some additional arguments that they had not previously considered. Those who disagree on the basis of sound arguments of their own will of course not be dissuaded by my comments; but they may achieve a greater appreciation of the vulnerable points in their own case, where stronger arguments may be necessary to buttress it.

Nuclear Arms

Having recently been part of an effort to secure the sponsorship of various state and local medical societies for a proposed conference on the medical consequences of the nuclear arms race, I can testify to the ubiquity of one objection to physicians' having a role in the nuclear debate—that medicine and politics don't mix, and that the nuclear issue is clearly a political one, not a medical, scientific, or educational one. One member of the county medical society put the conflict in stark form: "If I had wanted to go into politics, I wouldn't have gone into medicine."

To deny that any discussion of the medical and scientific aspects of the nuclear arms race and the threat of nuclear holocaust has major political overtones would simply be disingenuous. Here, once more, an originally neutral word has in modern usage acquired a derogatory connotation. When our elected representatives choose a course of action or inaction marked by unfair advantage being bestowed upon one petty interest group, we sneeringly describe the outcome as "politics as usual"; and when our representatives put aside self-interest to take action for the broader public good, we grudgingly salute them for "rising above politics." Politics is thus rendered indistinguishable from plotting and partisanship.

All of us know, but may periodically need to be reminded, that "politics" may be used on a loftier plane to refer to the general practices by which human beings can live cooperatively within social institutions, and bend those institutions to human needs and ends. We also know that the "either-or" approach to being a physician or being involved in politics is regrettably naive—as that speaker's very presence at the meeting of the county medical society tended to indicate. Local medical societies, hospital committees, and public health departments are political institutions, and few see it as contradicting the physician's fundamental identity to be involved in them.

The natural rejoinder is that "medical politics" is all right, but that the physician is stepping out of bounds to get involved in national politics if he or she has no special expertise on the issues.[4] Given the occasional arrogance of some physicians, who expect that their advice on any matter will automatically be accepted merely by virtue of the magic letters "MD" after their name, this modesty may at first seem commendable. Several observations raise questions about this reason not to get involved. First, a physician may offer public counsel on a political question without adopting the arrogant posture just criticized. If an insurance salesman gets up at a town meeting and presents his views on the proposed sewer system, we do not automatically assume that "he thinks we ought to believe what he says just because he's an insurance salesman," unless something in his manner or his wording forces this conclusion upon us; we give him the benefit of the doubt and assume that he hopes that the reasonableness of his supporting evidence will win us to his point of view, independent of his professional identity. Second, physicians are supposed to be concerned with the health and disease of their patients, which in turn implies an interest in the health or disease level of the entire community. Various political decisions may produce an increased risk of ill health; and furthermore, these decisions might be such that the individual actions of a single physician or a single patient will be ineffective in responding to them. In instances of a public health hazard, the physician must either give up his concerns over the health of his patients with regard to that risk factor, or else resign himself to involvement in the political process (either personally, or professionally via his representatives in various professional organizations).[5-7]

Finally, one consideration is peculiarly applicable to the nuclear issue. The "I'm not an expert so I can't get politically involved" argument implies the willingness to turn all relevant political decisions over to those who do claim to be experts. Social critics such as Illich and Lasch have pointed out the dangers of being too quick to unload all our social problems in this manner.[8,9] All physicians should be very sensitive to this point—after all, we are under increasing criticism for our supposed willingness to turn all human problems of living into medical problems, so that today's average citizen lives in mortal fear that some great evil will befall him unless he consults his doctor before eating, breathing, copulating, dying, or performing any other natural function that used to be taken for granted. We are starting to see in the medical journals editorial warnings about the "over-medicalization" of our culture, and most of us feel that it is about time. Therefore, we ought to be equally skeptical about the over-Pentagonization of everything that has to do with the nuclear arms race and planning for nuclear war. If in fact the data about nuclear strategy and the nature and potential uses of modern weapons systems were so arcane as to require years of study to master, physicians might be forgiven for abandoning the task; but when reading only a few sources (such as those cited in this chapter) provides a sufficient understanding of contemporary nuclear thinking to reveal some significant logical inconsistencies in our government's approaches to deterrence and arms control, failing to call attention frankly to these gaps and to demand reasonable answers from those in power amounts to agreeing to pretend that the emperor is wearing clothes. When (as Scheer describes) the person with the most significant national responsibility for civil-defense planning in the event of nuclear war contends that all the health effects of nuclear explosions can be mitigated simply by having everyone dig a hole, cover it with a door, pile dirt on top, and crawl into it, then any physician who does not object to this gross mockery of emergency preparedness is every bit as responsible as our profession would have been had we not raised questions about the safety and efficacy of Laetrile in cancer.[10]

All these considerations assume, of course, that those offering the no-expertise-so-no-politics excuse are not simply being hypocritical, approving of medical involvement in political issues that they favor and objecting only when they personally disagree with the politics. One may legitimately question their motives when one observes that at the same time that this "political" furor was being raised about the nuclear issue, the medical political action committees (PACs) had been second only to the real estate PACs in amount of money spent to influence Congressional elections in the previous election year.

THE PUBLIC HEALTH RESPONSIBILITY ARGUMENT

Cassel and Jameton have attempted to justify the physician's social responsibility for the nuclear war issue by making an analogy between the prevention of nuclear war and the prevention of other public health risks.[3] In order to judge the validity of their argument, and to see how well the analogy holds between nuclear war and other public health risks, it will be useful to restate their argument in outline form, using "X" as a temporary place-holder. The argument then is as follows:

1. Physicians have a special and central responsibility to treat disease and reduce mortality.
2. X would produce death or morbidity on a significant scale.
3. Once X has actually occurred, physicians could not intervene effectively to reduce the morbidity and mortality; their intervention would be considerably less effective than preventive efforts undertaken before X had occurred.
4. The occurrence of X is probable in the immediate future.
5. Physicians' efforts could be effective in preventing X.
6. Therefore, physicians have a special and central responsibility to work to prevent X.

Physicians in general are comfortable with this form of argument when X is replaced by "a polio epidemic" or other widespread but preventable occurrences of infectious diseases. Consider other social evils that have been proposed as substitutes for X over the years—the deleterious effects on child health and development of laws that permit child labor; child abuse and neglect; teenage pregnancy; and antisocial behavior caused by watching too much television. It seems clear from these examples that a wide variety of human activities and natural events have been viewed as legitimate X's despite potential controversy over the degree of physician expertise regarding the X and the ability of physicians, acting alone, to do anything about X. The argument fails, of course, if medical expertise is insufficient to persuade the general public or the policymakers on points #2 and #3.

The argument will also fail if X turns out to have important social value for nonmedical reasons, such that the predicted benefits of X outweigh the predicted mortality and morbidity. This is an important consideration and one that is especially susceptible to miscalculation owing to physician arrogance or inappropriate generalization of expertise—that is, physicians may be so narrowly focused on the ill health effects of X as to be unable to perceive its great public benefits. In order to make sure that this sort of inappropriate physician arrogance is not inserted into the argument (a particular concern, as was noted previously, with the nuclear war issue), it might be appropriate to amend the Cassel-Jameton argument by inserting a new condition 6°, as follows:

1. Physicians have a special and central responsibility to treat disease and reduce mortality.
2. X would produce death or morbidity on a significant scale.
3. Once X has actually occurred, physicians could not intervene effectively to reduce the morbidity and mortality; their intervention would be considerably less effective than preventive efforts undertaken before X had occurred.
4. The occurrence of X is probable in the immediate future.
5. Physicians' efforts could be effective in preventing X.
6.° There is no compensating public benefit deriving from X such that the benefit outweighs the predicted mortality and morbidity.
7.° Therefore, physicians have a special and central responsibility to work to prevent X.

The importance of this additional condition in the medical debate over nuclear war is discussed presently. First, it may be helpful to assess exactly how compelling is the nuclear war-epidemic analogy, by following Cassel and Jameton in their point-by-point discussion of the other conditions.

1. The responsibility of physicians for the treatment and amelioration as well as the prevention of disease seems uncontroversial. The important point to note in connection with this argument is that this responsibility, in public health matters, extends also to educating the general public to the existence of the risks to health, if there are reasonable grounds to assume that the public at large may be insufficiently aware of them. Another way of putting this point is that if indeed the public at large is fully aware of the risks to health, but takes no action to remove X, there is reason to fear that condition 6° has not been met—that there is a compensating benefit resulting from X of which the public is fully aware but that the medical profession has chosen to ignore. Thus, a reasonable campaign for public education and awareness is crucial in establishing the validity of the entire argument.

2. The data to suggest the massive mortality and morbidity that would result from a nuclear holocaust have been compellingly presented in the medical literature by Ervin et al 20 years ago and more recently by Abrams and von Kaenel.[11,12] Representative figures from the latter authors (assuming a 6500-megaton attack upon the United States, a moderate use of weapons as the current nuclear arsenals go) include: 86 million killed and 34 million injured in the first hour after the attack; an additional 50 million deaths in the next four weeks, the so-called shelter period; and between one and six months after the attack, an additional 15 million deaths from one single cause alone—the predicted epidemics of infectious disease resulting from a combination of specially favorable circumstances (from the microbe's point of view) that would be a function of the postattack environment. These

figures, as ballpark estimates, have not been questioned by any of the medical organizations, such as the American Academy of Pediatrics, the American College of Physicians, and the American Medical Association, which have adopted resolutions on nuclear war.[13]

As depressing as such figures may be, they may tell only the smaller part of the story of the consequences of an all-out nuclear attack. Projections of studies such as that of the Royal Swedish Academy of Sciences in their journal *Ambio*, based on data that have been summarized in a very readable and compelling form by Schell, raise questions of whether the global ecosystem, following a nuclear holocaust, would be able to support human life in any form at all, or whether the effects of fallout, increased ultraviolet penetration owning to destruction of the ozone layer, and global climatic alterations would not produce the eventual extinction of all surviving humans, as well as the extinction of many other plant and animal species.[1,14] While the actual likelihood of these global effects defies precise prediction, the fact that they cannot scientifically be excluded from possibility or even probability suggests that the early mortality and morbidity figures of the medical projections, as horrible as they are, may be almost irrelevant to the issue. Cassel and Jameton recognize this additional dimension of the problem. They engage in a quantitative exercise in an effort to calculate the probability of a nuclear war occurring in the next 20 years that would yield a number of expected deaths equal to the number of deaths from cancer in the same period—the point being that if nuclear war is seen as being at least that probable (their conclusion is, between one in 20 and one in 50), physicians ought to devote at least as much effort and concern to the prevention of nuclear war as we now devote to the "war" on cancer. They acknowledge that this calculation treats nuclear holocaust as an event on a par with cancer, however—as something that may produce much death and disability, but that does not in itself threaten the very survival of our culture, our society, and our species. Once the possible global ecologic effects are taken into account, "this possibility raises concern about nuclear war to a moral level at which cost-benefit analysis is meaningless and utterly absurd."[3]

3. The medical projections emphasize the woefully inadequate medical response that could be expected in a postattack environment. Abrams and von Kaenel project an 80% casualty rate among health professionals, leaving each surviving physician with 177 acutely injured survivors requiring treatment, in the absence (in all likelihood) of any electrical power, transportation, communication, hospital facilities, laboratories, x-ray facilities, drugs, or vaccines.[11] Other estimates are more pessimistic, projecting 1700 injured victims for each surviving physician.[11,15,16] Lest these figures be seen as mere scare tactics, it is worth contemplating the estimates of the one organization that expresses optimism over the ability of our society to survive a nuclear attack, the Federal Emergency Management Administration (FEMA). FEMA officials have testified before Congress that under the most favorable circumstances (which include full funding of all FEMA projects, a three-

to-eight-day warning of a possible attack, and full cooperation of the general public with every aspect of a massive evacuation scheme), 80% of the population of the US might be expected to survive.

Let us for one minute grant all the extravagant assumptions required to make this outcome plausible, and look simply at the 80% figure. This seems to suggest that 20% would not survive; and this 20% currently consists of 45 million Americans. For purposes of comparison, look up "Disasters" in a standard almanac and add up the total number of persons killed in all of the great disasters of history. Using a recent edition of the *Information Please Almanac* and a pocket calculator, I derived the figure of 4.4 million. We are thus presented with this interesting result—that according to the *most optimistic* estimates anyone dares to make, the number of deaths in the US resulting from a nuclear attack will be *ten times* the number of deaths resulting from the total of all the great disasters in this history of the world. This single statistic should drive home both the extent of mortality to be expected from nuclear war, and the inability of the medical community to make any meaningful impact on the outcome. (Under ordinary circumstances, medical measures that can be expected to result in the saving of twenty million lives would appear to be a tremendous accomplishment. If we set our nation on a course that risks a nuclear war, however, in which the lives of 40 million citizens will be lost, it seems to require a very perverted value system to take any solace at all in the observation that had we not engaged in some sort of medical preparedness planning, 60 million people would have died instead. It also requires a value system that discounts totally the loss of lives in other countries besides the US.)

4. Cassel and Jameton use a one-in-20 chance that a nuclear war will occur in the remaining years of this century as a conservative estimate. Many authorities place the odds at nearer to certainty unless there is a major change in the momentum of the nuclear arms race. It is worth recalling that in one recent 18-month period, there were approximately 150 human or computer errors in the US radar defense system, any one of which, if not detected in time, could have resulted in a US counterattack to a nonexistent Soviet first strike.[1]

5. The rapid increase in membership and influence of groups such as the Physicians for Social Responsibility, and the increasing attention to the nuclear war issue in both the medical journals and the lay press, tend to support the proposition that physicians, while they cannot unilaterally halt the arms race, can have a significant effect on public awareness and public attitudes. Certainly, the various medical organizations and specialty societies mentioned previously that have adopted nuclear-war resolutions have some degree of faith in the power of medical opinion to command a sympathetic hearing.

As has been argued, conditon number 6° is necessary to the argument in order to avoid the unacceptable physician arrogance of claiming to weigh competing values on behalf of society as a whole. It is precisely with the inclusion of this condition, however, that the argument demonstrates the impossibility of avoiding a political debate when the physician's responsibility for the prevention of nuclear war is discussed. The question must unavoidably arise whether the construction of nuclear weapons and the continued threat to use nuclear weapons do not serve a much greater social purpose—the defense of our country—so as to override any concern for negative health consequences. This is especially true if defenders of the policy of deterrence and negotiation from strength (like Huth in the medical press) are justified in their assumptions that it is only through escalating and continuing the nuclear arms race that we render it unlikely that a nuclear war will occur.[17] It is quite true that the prediction of the likelihood of nuclear confrontation given various international scenarios is far removed from the training and expertise of the average physician. Nevertheless, I do not see how the matter can be avoided entirely in medical discussions of this issue. I believe that the references listed at the end of the chapter give a reasonable overview of this issue and provide compelling reasons to fear that the threat of nuclear war growing out of the mere continuation of the nuclear arms race and the present international stalemate far outweighs any imagined security that the accumulation of weapons of destruction provides for our nation. The argument that a strong nuclear arsenal is our best defense against the possibility of nuclear war makes this simplistic assumption that the major nuclear danger comes from a willful decision on the part of one of our international adversaries to launch a nuclear attack against us. The argument neglects completely the possibility of accidental nuclear war due to human failure or computer error; the more nuclear weapons that are accumulated and the more complex the technology that controls them, the greater this likelihood appears. Physicians concerned with nuclear issues must address the current public delusion that the accumulation of more nuclear weapons makes us more safe rather than less safe, in much the same way that we would try to counter the widespread public belief that one is safe driving a car if one does not use seatbelts or child safety restraints (despite the fact that physicians are not experts in automotive engineering).

ISSUES OF SPECIAL CONCERN IN CHILDREN AND ADOLESCENTS

All the arguments in the preceding section apply equally to all physicians regardless of specialty. A few considerations, however, suggest that the issues raised are of particular interest to practitioners whose primary concern is with the health of children and adolescents.

When the nuclear issue is discussed among pediatricians, one sometimes hears the remark that the body of a child is much more sensitive to effects of ionizing radiation, and the other medical consequences of nuclear weapons, then are adults. On further analysis however, this argument does not seem to have significance in proving that pediatricians have any special responsibility for the issue of nuclear arms. The very gloomy predictions about the possibility of survival after a nuclear attack, given the total disruption of the social fabric, economic productivity, and medical capacity to treat the victims, render it likely in general that the survival of one threat to health merely means that one becomes a potential victim of the next line of disastrous long-range consequences. With regard to all the possible ways that one can be killed as a result of nuclear war, being a child or being an adult seems to make about as much difference in long-term survival and health outlook as would the difference between being in the front line or the rear guard among Custer's troops at the Battle of the Little Big Horn.

Another issue, however, is of particular concern to those caring for children and youth. This is the question of the massive amounts of societal resources that are currently devoted to the arms race, and which could be spent in much more healthful ways to promote the best interest of our younger citizens, especially among the poorer and disadvantaged classes. Hiatt has argued this point persuasively in the medical literature.[18] Given that children and youth are in a position of relative political powerlessness to defend their own special interests, especially when poverty is added as a disadvantage, they are a tempting group from which financial resources can be diverted once it is decided that more money is needed to fuel the nuclear arms race. In viewing the importance of this particular argument, it should be noted that not everyone who opposes the nuclear arms race and the possible use of nuclear weapons is necessarily a pacifist and would desire that any money saved from the reduction in our nuclear arsenals would automatically be used for social welfare purposes. A number of the most vocal opponents of current US nuclear policy have made the point that the United States has leaned too heavily on nuclear arsenals while allowing our conventional defense forces to deteriorate markedly. This group feels that there is legitimate reason to fear Soviet imperialism in Europe, for example, if the United States disarms on the nuclear side without a corresponding increase in conventional weaponry. Accordingly, their argument is for nuclear disarmament, but with diversion of the money saved to conventional weapons for a stronger national defense. If this argument is the one that eventually prevails in the political arena, it will not be the case that nuclear disarmament will necessarily mean more money for health care programs. However, to the extent that the financial resources needed to accelerate the arms race are presently being diverted from other categories of social spending, the consequences for all segments of society, including the young, definitely should be assessed and spelled out explicitly.

Finally, there is the issue of the psychologic burden of the threat of nuclear war in the minds of children and adolescents. Unpublished surveys by Drs. William Beardslee and John Mack demonstrate a widespread degree of awareness of the dangers of nuclear war and an accompanying mood of fear and hopelessness among school children of diverse ages. The possibility that a good deal of childhood depression, psychologic trauma, and perhaps antisocial and delinquent behavior can in some way be linked to the nuclear concerns of children cannot be lightly dismissed. In our adult society, we can perhaps continue to deny the ever-present threat of nuclear annihilation while we swear allegiance to a government that continues to increase the risks of this annihilation by its actions, and consider ourselves sophisticated and emotionally mature because we can engage in this sort of double-think. Children and adolescents are generally much less able to live with contradictions of this sort without undergoing severe psychic distress. It remains to be seen whether the children who would demand that we confront this contradiction in our society are not more mature and realistic that we adults who think we can avert our gaze.

CONCLUSION: A RESOLUTION ON NUCLEAR WAR

Whereas,—the American Academy of Pediatrics has steadfastly maintained its advocacy for the health, safety and well-being of the children of the Americas for more than a half a century; and

Whereas,—a nuclear war would wreak long-term catastrophic effects on present and future generations of children everywhere, effects which the medical community would be powerless to treat adequately; and

Whereas,—the medical community has an obligation to make public comment on the medical aspects of this vital issue and to arouse its members and the general public to the dangers and implications of nuclear warfare; be it

RESOLVED,—that the American Academy of Pediatrics communicate its concern about the medical effects of a nuclear war to appropriate public and private organizations, including the President and Congress, and that it inform its membership of the dire consequences of nuclear war.

American Academy of Pediatrics, Executive Board Minutes Appendix 13, June 1982.

REFERENCES

1. Schell: The Fate of the Earth. New York, Alfred A. Knopf, 1982.
2. Jonsen AR: On Being a Casuist. Paper presented at the Conference on Clinical Medical Ethics: Exploration and Assessment, Knoxville, TN, August 16, 1982.
3. Cassel C, Jameton A: Medical Responsibility and Thermonuclear War. Ann Intern Med 97:426–432, 1982.
4. Relman S: Physicians, Nuclear War, and Politics. N Engl J Med 307:744–745, 1982.
5. Brody H: The Family Physician and Nuclear War. J Family Prac 15:371–372, 1982.

6. Lown B, et al: The Nuclear-Arms Race and the Physician. N Engl J Med 304:726–729, 1981.
7. Neal E: Nuclear Weapons and War: The Transcendent Health Problem. J Family Prac 14:647–649, 1982.
8. Illich I: Medical Nemesis. New York, Pantheon, 1976.
9. Lasch C: The Culture of Narcissism. New York, WW Norton, 1979.
10. Scheer R: With Enough Shovels: Reagan, Bush and Nuclear War. New York, Random House, 1982.
11. Ervin FR, et al: The Medical Consequences of Thermonuclear War. N Engl J Med 266:1126–1155, 1962.
12. Abrams HL, Von Kaenel WE: Medical Problems of Survivors of Nuclear War. N Engl J Med 305:1226–1232, 1981.
13. Health Policy Committee, American College of Physicians: The Medical Consequences of Radiation Accidents and Nuclear War. Ann Intern Med 97:447–450, 1982.
14. Nuclear War: The Aftermath. Ambio (J Human Environment, Royal Swedish Academy of Sciences), Volume II, Number 2–3, 1982.
15. Adams R, Cullen S (eds): The Final Epidemic: Physicians and Scientists on Nuclear War. Chicago, Educational Foundation for Nuclear Science, 1981.
16. Chivian E, et al (eds): Last Aid: The Medical Dimensions of Nuclear War. San Francisco, WH Freeman, 1982.
17. Huth EJ: The Road Away from Nuclear War. Ann Intern Med 97:445–446, 1982.
18. Hiatt HH: The Physician and National Security. N Engl J of Med 307:1142–1145, 1982.

C. Richard Cornelius, J.D.

20

LEGAL ISSUES IN PEDIATRIC PRACTICE

It is clear that the law today touches all aspects of health care. This phenomenon has developed slowly through the course of the twentieth century, with a precipitate increase in medical-legal matters occurring during the past decade. Although many physicians would consider it of dubious distinction, the sheer genius and energies of medicine and technology over the past quarter century have encouraged and required closer legal inquiry into medicine. The law in most situations merely reflects the will and decency norm of society. Thus, the law reacts to, checks, and balances the human experience.

Traditionally, physicians and lawyers have looked upon each other suspiciously. The advent of what euphemistically was referred to as the "malpractice crisis" of the mid 1970s has simply exasperated the relationship between these two professions. This chapter does not outline the origins of these strained relationships, nor does it suggest threads of common agreement and interest that could lessen this gulf of mistrust and hostility.

Instead, this chapter intends to enumerate and discuss legal principles that are part of each physician's practice. Since this book is dedicated to the treatment of children, the laws examined deal with those concepts that bear directly upon the pediatrician's practice. Obviously, certain concepts are relevant to medicine in general and to all health care providers. These concepts are listed and reviewed.

This article, therefore, undertakes: (1) an exploration of the law in general and the functioning of the court in particular, (2) a summary of the legal theory of malpractice coupled with advice on how to avoid its occurrence, (3) an approach to the substantive legal issues of pediatric practice, (4) the appropriate response to subpoenas and to the request for medical records, and (5) an analysis of the legal status of controversial aspects of the treatment of children.

UNDERTAKING THE LAW

The Working of the Court

Law adjudicates disputes, sets rights and responsibilities, and allows continuity for prospective decision-making in establishing precedents. Legislators, both federal and state, create the laws, while the courts interpret the law in regard to specific cases.

Medical professionals seem to be more aware of the legislative and political process. This is perhaps so because national medical organizations such as the American Medical Association, American College of Surgeons, and the American Academy of Pediatrics have long been interested in ensuring that the medical side is clearly presented and well represented in health care legislation. It is the court system, however, that presents more of a mystery to the health care professional, particularly the physician.

Going to court is mystifying, unpredictable, and therefore terrifying. Good trial lawyers will warn all would-be litigants of the traumas of testifying in a courtroom. Litigation is costly in more ways than dollars and cents.

Legal proceedings will always be a bit mysterious to the lay witness. Most lawyers will confess some confusion at times with court rulings, so it is not surprising that the testifying health professional should be concerned by the mysteries of the courtroom drama. Mystery and intrigue should not lead to fear or trepidation of the courtroom. Why so?

Legal trials involve both issues of law and questions of fact. The lawyers concern themselves with the legal issues, the jury and witness with the facts. When a health professional is called to testify, the court and the jury are there to listen to the health care provider tell the story. Although both court and jury must understand the testimony, the witness is conversing in his or her mother tongue—the language and experience of the professional. It is thus not a situation where the witness is a fish out of water. More often than not, the witness is educating the court in the ways and intricacies of his or her profession. Obviously, the better versed and informed one is in his profession, the easier it is to testify clearly, confidently, and securely.

The medical malpractice case is a fine example of how, at least in theory, the medical professional and profession can and do help control outcome.

Four critical issues face the court in each and every medical malpractice case. In each issue, the burden of proof rests with the plaintiff or complainant in order to establish the case. These issues are:

1. Establishing the standard of care in the medical community—what is the customary practice of similar practitioners in the field?
2. Proving that the defendant health care provider has failed in this case to maintain the accepted standard or norm of care. Here the complainant must establish that the health care professional has deviated abnormally from the standard.
3. Complainant must establish that the direct act(s) that deviate from the accepted standard(s) (the negligence or malpractice) have *caused* the injury or damages to the complainant.
4. The complainant has suffered fixed and predictable injuries and damages as a direct result of the health care professional's acts of bad practice.

In each of these four issues, the health care professional plays the dominant role in formulating the answers. Without the testimony of credentialed experts in the health sciences, none of these issues could be resolved satisfactorily by the court or the jury. Therefore, it is not the law, the judge, or the jury that establishes medical standards or acceptable practices, but rather health care professionals themselves who tell the court what the standards are. These standards are not established on whim or possibility, knowing full well that almost everything is possible. Health care professionals who testify as experts can only render opinions or conclusions that are based upon reasonable degrees of medical probabilities or certainties.

These are not weak or frivolous tests which the complainant must pass. Each test calls for demonstrating and proving tangible evidence that is more persuasive than that shown by the defending health care professional. The complainant cannot succeed without the support of the medical community through use of expert medical testimony and reliance upon the wealth of medical journals, texts, and treatises. It is this message, then, that can be left with the health care professionals: They and their professions play a significantly critical and dominant role in establishing the standards that guide and carve out legal opinions. If this be the case, the health care professional called to testify should not fear, for all that is required is the ability to communicate and to teach the lay judge and jury something about what he or she practices and experiences professionally on a daily basis. If testifying can be reduced to this objective, the conscientious health care professional will have no problem when his day in court arrives.

LEGAL THEORY OF MEDICAL MALPRACTICE

In 1973, it was recognized by the American Academy of Pediatrics that pediatricians were generally ill informed about basic medical-legal issues. In that year, a task force of the Academy was created to examine the medical liability issues as they impacted upon the pediatrician. This self-help process did not begin too soon. Since 1973, pediatricians have seen the first medical malpractice crisis. Most legal and insurance commentators talk of a new crisis just around the corner. Malpractice judgments and settlements continue to skyrocket to levels that are well beyond the significant mark. Whether these levels are reasonable or patently absurd is of little relevance, since the judgments and settlements continue to increase in numbers and amounts. Of course, this trend is relevant and has far-reaching impact on the medical and legal professions. However, to judge the fairness or societal worth of these numbers is irrelevant in that the cases and amounts awarded are real and must be observed and heeded by each practicing pediatrician. Simply speaking, ignoring the subject or lamenting its impact on the practice of medicine is useless and dangerous to the practitioner. However, certain steps can be taken in each practice to minimize the chances of a lawsuit from a disgruntled patient and his family.

Although 1973 seems to be the year of awareness for the Academy of Pediatrics, legal cases had by then long since established principles which would guide the development and prosecution of the medical malpractice case as it is known today.

Medical malpractice law comes under the general heading of tort law. A tort, a word of latin etymology, stands for conduct that is twisted or not straight. Broadly used, a tort is a civil wrong not involving contracts for which courts provide legal remedies in the form of monetary damages.[1] This form of legal action originated in the early part of the nineteenth century. The law of torts establishes standards of conduct in the various fields. A person who does not meet "the standard in so doing breaches the standard and may be liable." The word "negligence" has become synonymous with torts. A person who breaches the standard is negligent. In fact, this use of the "professions" was an early development of this American law of torts. Concepts of negligence and liability were developed by those who professed to be skilled and versed in "public" callings, such as surgeons.[2]

A tort cause of action requires the presence of certain elements in order to succeed. First, a legal duty or obligation exists requiring activity that will not cause unreasonable risks to the public and that involves standard of conduct or standard of care. This principle is very much in evidence in all things a professional does. In order to practice the arts and skills of a profession, the actor must conform to rudimentary skills, tasks, and criteria. As an example, in the practice of pediatrics, it is a universal recognized standard to recommend to the parents of newborns the importance of vaccine immunization for childhood diseases.

Second, there must be failure on the part of the professional to conform to the required standard. Third, a proximate relation to or "legal cause" between the aberrant conduct and the injury to the third party or person must exist. Fourth, and finally, actual damage to the third party's interests must occur.

Returning to our immunization example, it is easy to see how a pediatrician becomes liable to the child and parents when he fails to provide immunization and the child contracts a childhood disease which is today avoidable through immunization.

Now that the legal theory of medical malpractice has been presented, what can the pediatrician do to avoid its occurrence?

1. Seriously consider the importance of complete, objective, and logically sound documentation that is contemporaneous with the medical device used and procedure performed (see later).
2. Do not overlook or treat hastily the process of informing the patient and family about medical treatments and procedures (see later—discussion of informed consent).
3. Maintain all medical records in conformance with state laws on the age of majority plus appropriate Statute of Limitations period.
4. Obtain reasonable and realistic medical malpractice insurance coverage, preferably on an occurrence as opposed to a claims-made basis.
5. Do not overlook the need for subspecialty evaluation on a consultative basis to achieve diagnostic confirmation. The corollary rule also applies; encourage and certainly do not discourage the patient/family from obtaining second opinions when they wish or broach the subject.

THE SUBSTANTIVE LEGAL ISSUES OF PEDIATRIC PRACTICE

An all-too-brief general presentation of legal issues involving pediatric practice is all that can be expected in a brief chapter. Listing most of the legal areas that the pediatrician will face in a daily practice can be instructive for no other reason than to demonstrate dramatically the law's influence upon medicine. Although each subject listed is worthy of and requires at least a chapter in itself, two subjects demand more attention. It is the author's belief that the health care professional's basic understanding of medical records documentation and informed consent principles are the two most important "legal" considerations that warrant understanding and attention in the daily practice of medicine.

PROPER MEDICAL RECORDS DOCUMENTATION

Informative charting should be a timely and timeless subject for all health professionals. Whether properly taught or not in the medical and nursing schools, the art of charting often is lost in daily practice. From a legal perspective, the poorly charted record, often incomplete and judgmental, can bring about the undoing of the health professional, whose acts may later be scrutinized by a jury. In such situations, the poorly recorded chart can become a rather efficient weapon with which the plaintiff's lawyer can cast suspicions on the acts of the defending nurses and physicians.

In short, other than the witness' own credibility, no piece of evidence is more crucial in a medical malpractice trial than the medical record of the complaining patient. For this reason alone, the medical record must be informative. It must accurately and completely describe the patient's condition and each treatment administered. In malpractice litigation, the jury invariably places trust in the veracity of the written medical record, thus making it all the more important to enter each medical course of action. Experience has shown that a jury will rarely believe the oral testimony of medical personnel if it deviates from data entered in the medical record. Oral testimony may serve to confirm the medical record; rarely, however, will it persuade a jury when the medical record offers conflicting information.

Most dangerous from a defense perspective are those records that include judgmental remarks or subjective conclusions. The off-service "good luck" note from the retiring resident to the oncoming team is one example; another is the far too common practice of using ambivalent terms like "inappropriate" or "difficult" to describe the conduct of a parent or guardian without further explanation.

One additional suggestion relating to informative and effective medical record charting is the use of the cosignature as witness to psychosocial behavioral incidents concerning the patient and family members. Corroborative testimony is the stuff of which successful defensive suits are made.

Medical records are readily available, admissible, and compelling evidence to the jury. Regardless of the optimal quality of care given, incomplete charting may place the good practitioner in an indefensible position. The excuse of the practitioner that he or she does not have time to document is a lame and inexcusable rationale for leaving gaps in medical documentation.

INFORMED CONSENT

Perhaps no legal theory has engendered more controversy, resentment, or misunderstanding within the medical community than the doctrine of informed consent. Its genesis can be traced to dicta in a 1920 legal opinion written by former Supreme Court Justice Benjamin Cardozo; however, 40 more years would elapse before the doctrine gained full recognition in American jurisprudence.[3,4]

Informed consent is based upon the belief that every person has the right to determine what shall be done with his or her body. This right is not surrendered when one seeks a physician for medical advice.[5] To fulfill this right, the patient must have sufficient information to make an "informed" choice, and then "consent" to or authorize a particular medical treatment.

If the medical community is reluctant to accept the doctrine, it is primarily because they perceive it as one more societal intrusion upon an already beleaguered professional practice, not because they question the premise upon which it is based. Many doctors inform (instruct) their patients routinely concerning the nature of proposed treatment, irrespective of legal pronouncements on the subject. These physicians would readily conclude that a sound physician-patient relationship depends largely on such disclosures.

Not one court or case has yet sanctioned the use of a general consent or authorization form that does not require the physician to elaborate specific risks or alternatives.[6] In fact, the courts have termed general forms as worthless and, without more proof or evidence that an informed consent was obtained, as ineffective defense that the medical procedure was performed subsequent to an intelligent assent by the patient. The law is thus demanding substance over "the form."

This is not to say that the general consent form is useless. Such forms, which relate primarily to history-taking, physician examinations, diagnostic work-ups, and medication, have become an integral part of inpatient and outpatient admissions procedures. The general form should be, however, an administrative responsibility, and not the concern of the physician.

The law demands that information of a more specific nature be conveyed by a physician in order to obtain an informed consent of the type that would be valid in situations involving surgical or medical procedures requiring anesthesia. Information that must be explained to the patient or parent in a pediatric setting includes:

1. physician's diagnosis;
2. general nature of the proposed treatment;
3. risks involved in the proposed treatment;
4. prospects of success;
5. prognosis if the procedure is not performed; and
6. any reasonable alternative methods of treatment.

Anything short of this would not constitute an informed consent. Furthermore, in addition to the six-step explanation just outlined, most courts will determine the adequacy of the disclosure by relying upon a "materiality test," ie, the disclosure must include whatever information is material to the patient's decision, whether or not the patient asks for such information.

Furthermore, the courts have recognized three definite exceptions to the requirement of full disclosure in informed consent cases. The "medical emergency"; the "ignorance is bliss" situation, in which the patient states that he or she would prefer to remain ignorant of the potential complications of a procedure; and the "peace of mind" case, in which the patient's psyche requires less than full disclosure.[7-9] Neither of the latter two exceptions would be suitable defenses for the pediatrician.

Fully armed with knowledge of the law, how can the physician best prevent legal action based upon an informed consent theory? Certainly there is nothing sacrosanct about a written, as opposed to an oral, consent. Both are legal and sufficient; however, legal actions rise or fall on the physical availability and persuasiveness of the evidence. A parent's claim that he or she was not fully informed before assenting to treatment of the child may convince the jury, when the sole *contra* evidence is the physician's testimony, that the parent was informed. This clearly is not a legally ideal situation for the defense.

Consent forms are not ideal either; however, a clearly written, specific "Consent to Surgical, Anesthesia, or Special Medical Procedures" form can afford as much protection as possible. Obtaining written consent is the nondelegable responsibility of the physician, and it is imperative that the physician sign the consent form to show evidence of the explanation. Forms executed by office or hospital personnel are not legally acceptable. A witness should be present while the physician, the parent, and, when applicable, the child sign. It is not necessary, however, that the witness be present during the physician's explanation itself. The form must be easy to use; blanks should be filled in with specific information about the particular procedure in question.

In what detail and to what extent must risks and alternatives be disclosed? The law does not mandate "full" disclosure; instead, it requires a reasonable effort by the physician to identify clearly those factors that could materially affect the patient's decision to undergo or forego a particular treatment. The physician is not obligated to discuss unforeseeable risks or complications "of which persons of average sophistication are aware."[10] Moreover, it would be ill advised to list every specific risk for each case. One may understandably forget to list a certain risk even though it had been discussed.

Informed consent poses unique problems to physicians who treat minors, for they must reakon with a second "patient," ie, the parent or guardian of the child. Society has recognized a legal and moral need for parents to authorize treatment, thereby substituting their best judgment for that of their minor children. Although such a situation has never been tested, it is unlikely that a court would accept the "ignorance is bliss" or "peace of mind" defenses in a pediatric case, for while the adult has the legal right not to be informed of the risks of a procedure for himself, this same right is not transferable to pediatric cases. A court would undoubtedly have little difficulty in concluding that there was not only a right to full disclosure with regard to their child's condition and proposed therapy, but also a nondelegable responsibility of the parent to know and be informed.

This situation obviously necessitates frankness between the pediatrician and parents in all cases, with the understanding that it may create psychologic burdens and anxiety for the parent. This burden is particularly apparent when the physician explains possible, but extremely unlikely, serious risks in the more "routine" cases. As an example, it is a harsh and improbable consequence of adenoidectomy, circumcision, or herniorrhaphy that airway obstruction or cardiac arrest during anesthesia might cause severe brain damage or death. These unlikely complications can occur, however, no matter how skillfully anesthesia is planned, performed, and managed. It is this circumstance, the routine elective procedure with an unusual complication, that may cause the unsuspecting physician the greatest problems in an informed consent case, for it is this same "routine" case in which the physician does not wish to alarm the parents unduly. Again, however unpleasant disclosure of possible risks may be, the law requires a frank discussion of the improbable, serious complications with the parents prior to their consent and authorization for treatment.

The legal doctrine of informed consent, although generally new in legal circles, is already firmly established in various degrees in most jurisdictions. It is here to stay. The medical community may understandably feel somewhat irritated by this additional legal intrusion. Upon close look, however, the doctrine merely restates and validates a time-honored practice followed by many physicians long before judicial scrutiny began. Moreover, documenting the disclosure, as well as beginning the dialogue early in the relationship, can go a long way toward preventing later misunderstandings, distrust, and disappointment—the ingredients of potential lawsuits. Good "bedside manners" may be the best common-sense guide to the physician in implementing a satisfactory consent procudure.

HANDLING THE INQUIRING ATTORNEY AND DEALING WITH THE SUBPOENA

Even if not sued directly, chances are that a physician, nurse, or other health care provider in a major clinical center or in private practice will at some time receive a subpoena. A subpoena is a legal document that requires the recipient to appear in court to give testimony. The receipt of a subpoena gives rise to a legal obligation on the part of the recipient.

Failure to obey a subpoena may be deemed contempt of court. Because of this, guidelines are offered to assist the health care provider in complying with the requirements of the subpoena. Since some subpoenas received by health care professionals solicit testimony involving child abuse cases, as an example, the following guidelines are discussed in that context.

1. Look at who signed the subpoena. Is the family requesting your testimony, or is the government or state attorneys?
2. Note the date and time of the hearing or trial when you are to appear as a witness. If you are unable to attend for a valid reason, contact the subpoenaing attorney.
3. The subpoena may indicate that medical records are needed. In this situation, the following steps should be taken:
   a. Review the medical record.
   b. Copy the pertinent parts. For an outpatient, these would include the treatment sheet and follow-up instructions. For an admission, these would include the face sheet, exam sheet, and progress notes.
   c. Keep the copies in your personal file.
   d. Call the prosecutor and ask if it is necessary to bring the whole medical record or if your copies of pertinent parts will suffice.
   e. If the entire medical record is required, bring it with you but make sure it is returned.
4. Following your testimony, make sure that you sign the payment of

witness fee and return medical records to the hospital. You should be compensated for your time. The fee will depend upon whether you testify as a factual or an expert witness.

One of the first things a medical malpractice attorney considering a lawsuit against a health care provider wants is the patient's medical record. Review of the record allows the plaintiff-patient's attorney to assess the merits of a possible claim. However, the unfortunate by-product of this phenomenon is an increasing number of requests to hospitals and physicians for copies of patient medical records. Frequently, letters of request are followed or preceded by phone calls from attorneys to physicians directly in an attempt to discuss the patient's care with the treating physician.

The physician or other health care provider may think that he or she is legally required to respond to such calls without scrutiny. However, this is not the case. In fact, health care providers can save themselves aggravation, time, and adverse legal outcomes by carefully handling attorneys' requests for records and telephone discussions regarding patient care.

Some recommend handling attorneys' requests for records as follows:

1. Letters from attorneys must be accompanied by proper authorization for release of information regarding the child's care signed by the parent or legal guardian.
2. Once received, and whether directed to the individual physician or to the hospital, such letters and the authorization are immediately forwarded to the Medical Records Department for processing.
3. The outside request should be complied with by the Medical Records Department or physician as directed. Any questions or concerns should be forwarded to legal counsel.
4. Telephone calls from attorneys to individual health care providers regarding patient records, or for that matter, any other patient-related medical/legal inquiry, should be avoided. While it may be tempting for the health care provider to reach for the phone just to "find out what the attorney wants," this is, without question, risky. The inquiring attorney may cleverly elicit information that later on could shift the tide of legal events against the health care provider.
5. When requests for records come from outside physicians, health care providers generally reasonably assume such requests to be without legal ramifications. However, our experience has shown that such requests may be not for the purpose of continuing medical treatment of the patient, but for the medical/legal review of the patient's past care. The requesting physician may be a possible expert witness hired by the plaintiff patient to help develop the malpractice case. Alternatively, he or she may be a physician attorney who is looking at the case from a legal standpoint. Know your physician!

LEGAL STATUS OF CARING FOR THE DEFECTIVE NEWBORN, HANDICAPPED CHILD, AND DYING PEDIATRIC PATIENT

These subjects have created the most controversial cases and provocative issues for the pediatric health care provider. Court precedent has been limited, statutory guidance in the pediatric setting almost nonexistent, and proposed federal government regulations unwelcomed generally by the health professional and institution.

The issues first took legal prominence in the *Karen Ann Quinlan* case.[11]

On April 15, 1975, nine days before her twenty-first birthday, Karen Ann Quinlan stopped breathing on two occasions. Each cessation lasted two to 15 minutes. She was admitted to a New Jersey hospital suffering from coma of unknown cause. Exhaustive tests and laboratory work were performed. A pulmonary internist was unable to "wean" her from the respirator; the attending neurologist concluded that she was in a chronic "vegetative" state characterized by decortication of the brain.

Nearly four months later, Miss Quinlan's parents became convinced that all medical assistance had been tried with no success and that continued use of the mechanical respirator to sustain life was not in Karen's best interest. The decision was made only after the parents had received extensive counseling and pastoral support. The hospital supported the family's decision. Karen's attending physician, however, was unwilling to comply with the parents' wishes. He refused to remove the respirator. The Quinlans initiated legal proceedings.

The Supreme Court of New Jersey ruled that the Quinlans had a legal right to seek the medical advice and ultimate opinion of a hospital ethics committee to determine the advisability of removing Karen from the respirator. The court further concluded that the use of a mechanical respirator to sustain life may be viewed in certain factual circumstances as extraordinary medical treatment that need not be administered indefinitely to certain dying or medically hopeless patients.

THE QUINLAN PROGENY

Both the medical community and society in general have benefited from the Quinlan opinion. Among the more important issues that it has brought to light is the necessity of a viable legal definition of death. The formulation of legal tests to determine the moment of death has, unfortunately, not kept pace with recent dramatic advances in medical technology. A number of states, for example, have legislated a brain-death standard modeled upon criteria published in 1968 by the Ad Hoc Committee of the Harvard Medical School. Simply stated, the Harvard test sets forth four basic criteria to define death: (1) unresponsiveness and unreceptiveness; (2) no movements or breathing; (3) no reflexes; and (4) flat EEG. Most jurisdictions recognize by law the Harvard criteria.

In spite of increasing focus on such matters in the wake of the Quinlan case, the case of the hopeless pediatric patient had not yet been confronted by our lawmakers and courts. This is perhaps in part because the decision to withdraw mechanical life support from a child is an especially wrenching and emotionally charged experience, since the child has not had the opportunity to live a full life. Moreover, there is no way in which to ascertain what choice the young patient would have made, had he or she been able to express an opinion.

The need for the medical and legal communities to face these issues was and still is urgent, for examples of the terminal or hopeless pediatric case are unfortunately endless—the child who has had a playground accident causing severe head trauma and irreversible brain damage, the child who nearly drowns, the acute leukemic, and the victim of overwhelming burns.

The Down's syndrome case aside, the use of the "No Code 99" or "No Code Blue" has now been accepted in most medical institutions as well as in the medical journals. Quinlan was not a "No Code" case per se, since her case involved the removal of life support treatment that had already been initiated. (The "No Code" case generally involves the decision to withhold life support treatment.) Despite this distinction, the same judicial principles and conclusions are applicable.

When "No Code" is used in the pediatric setting, certain standards must be observed by the institution and the administering physician to minimize the possibility of subsequent legal challenge. First, the attending physician must conduct a thorough medical examination. Specialists and subspecialists must examine the patient to corroborate the attending physician's findings. Careful documentation of all physicians' findings must then be charted in the patient's progress notes.

Second, the attending physician should have a frank, compassionate discussion of the child's condition with the parents or legal guardian. The critical importance of constant communication cannot be overemphasized. The specialist should also be called upon to provide support upon request. It is imperative that the parents appreciate the terminal nature of their child's condition and that they understand fully the appropriateness of the "No Code" order. The physician should take care to assure that the family is prepared both intellectually and emotionally to accept the consequences of their decision. If, after many hours of sensitive discussion, the parents concur that extraordinary treatment is not in the child's best interests, a "No Code" may be ordered. The conversation must be documented by the attending physician and should be witnessed.

Third, a "No Code" order should be written clearly and without equivocation in the child's chart. A misconception of no small proportion continues to surround this issue. It is important that it be fully understood that whether the "No Code" order is recorded or not will not alter: (1) the fact that the order was given; (2) its ultimate effect upon the patient and his or her family; and (3) the possibility of civil or criminal liability against the hospital or its employees for this decision.

There are, in fact, several distinct advantages, both legal and nonlegal, for documenting "No Code" decisions. From a nonlegal perspective, documentation is beneficial because it compels physicians to weigh carefully, after having received the advice of others, their course of action. Requiring documentation also guards against rash or indiscriminate use of the "No

Code" order. From a strictly legal point of view, the documentation protects the hospital and the attending physician from subsequent charges by the parents or third parties that the decision was inappropriate. The medical record reflects prior consultation with the parents and their participation in making the decision. Full responsibility for written documentation rests with the attending physician, thereby eliminating the possibility that nursing staff or other members of the health care team might be held accountable. It puts an end to possible charges of a conspiratorial "cover up." Failing to document such an action, on the other hand, may lend credence to the suspicion that "No Code" decisions result in an unethical or illegal procedure.

Following *Quinlan*, the recognition of brain death statutes, and the seeming acceptance of No Code decisions, the next front, and by far more controversial subject, is the treatment of the defective or profoundly handicapped infant. Again, this issue became front-page news following a decision by the Supreme Court of Indiana in *Baby Doe* of Bloomington, Indiana (unreported case).

In the Spring of 1982, a baby was born in Indiana with Down's syndrome and esophageal atresia that interfered with normal eating. His parents refused treatment for his medical problems and directed that intravenous feeding be withheld as well. The parents' decision was upheld by the Indiana Supreme Court, and soon thereafter the baby died. This is the latest of cases to appear in the press concerning infants born with severe deformity or illness whose parents, doctors, and ultimately the courts decide to treat or not treat.

Previously, when decisions whether to treat defective newborns were decided by courts, the trend was to order treatment. For example, within the past several years, courts in New York and Florida ordered the surgical treatment of two infants born with spina bifida over the parents' objections.[12,13]

However, one case that has reached the courts which is similar to the judicial outcome in the Indiana case is that of Phillip Becker in California.[14] Phillip was born with Down's syndrome and a heart defect. His parents opposed surgical correction of the heart defect and succeeded in obtaining the approval of the California Supreme Court in withholding this treatment. The Becker case is still pending on other technical legal grounds, and the ultimate outcome could differ. The Indiana and California cases, however, stand for the proposition that some courts may be increasingly willing to support nontreatment decisions. Certainly, both cases highlight a possible new judicial trend, and difficult issues will continue to develop in this area of health care law.

One such issue is whether treatment would have been more actively sought in these cases if the children had not been afflicted with Down's syndrome. Some commentators argue that it is the presence of Down's syndrome, or some other form of mental incapacity, that results in the decision not to treat in these cases, and that therefore the decision is a disguised quality of life call that possibly ought not be made in this manner.

Another issue centers on the type of treatment that is sought to be withheld. Decisions in the past have involved, for example, the withholding of surgery, mechanical respiratory assistance, and chemotherapy. Now, attention is being directed at situations in which more basic modes of medical management are sought to be withheld—for example, antibiotics. In fact, some characterize the Indiana Supreme Court decision as astonishing in that it marks the first time a court has approved the withholding of a very basic form of care, the intravenous feeding of an infant who because of the presence of esophageal atresia was unable to feed by mouth.

The records in the Bloomington case have been sealed, and therefore all the facts of that case are not available to the public. However, the case received enough attention to prompt President Reagan to send a memorandum to the Attorney General and to then-Secretary of Health and Human Services, Richard Schweiker, citing the "Baby Doe" case in Indiana and noting that federal law prohibits discrimination against the handicapped. In response to the President's memorandum, Secretary Schweiker issued a "notice" to health care providers to remind affected parties of the applicability of Section 504 of the Rehabilitation Act of 1973. This "notice" was issued on May 18, 1982 and was published in the Federal Register on June 16, 1982.

As further background, the President's Commission for the Study of Ethical Problems in Medicine and Biomedical and Behavioral Research completed a two-year intensive study of life-and-death issues in health care. This report was released on March 21, 1983, one day before publication of the "Interim Final Rule." That study gives a thoughtful and thorough report on the practice in health care institutions and offers realistic, workable suggestions that health care institutions can follow. The report recognized that there are instances in which it is appropriate to forego life-sustaining treatment for infants. It recommended that in making such decisions, parents receive complete relevant information, including as accurate an appraisal of prognosis as possible. It advised consultation with medical specialists, religious advisors, and other parents who have faced similar decisions. It recommended that enough time be allowed for thoughtful decision-making. The Commission recommended intrainstitutional review when appropriate and court-appointed surrogate guardians when parents are unable to reach a decision consistent with the child's best interests.

On Monday, March 7, 1983, the Secretary of Health and Human Services published an "Interim Final Rule" in the Federal Register. That rule noted that under Section 504 of the Rehabilitation Act of 1973, "no otherwise qualified handicapped individual . . . shall, solely by reason of his handicap, be excluded from participation in, be denied the benefits of, or be subjected to discrimination under any program or activity receiving federal financial assistance." Hospitals receiving federal financial assistance were required to post "in a conspicuous place in each delivery ward, each maternity ward, each pediatric ward, and each nursery, including each intensive care nursery," a sign containing this statement. The caption on the sign read:

DISCRIMINATORY FAILURE TO FEED AND CARE FOR HANDICAPPED INFANTS IN THIS FACILITY IS PROHIBITED BY FEDERAL LAW

The sign went on to state: Any person having knowledge that a handicapped infant is being discriminatorily denied food or customary medical care should immediately contact a "handicapped infant hotline."

The hotline call, which could be placed anonymously, would set into motion "Baby Doe Squads" which would immediately dispatch an investigatory team to the hospital to determine if, in fact, an infant's life was in danger because of "discriminatory care." This investigative team would have access to medical records and would interview staff and family to determine whether or not protective action was warranted.

On April 14, 1983, Judge Gerhard Gesell issued his decision in this case.[15] In invalidating the rule, the Judge based his decision on the government's violation of the Administrative Procedures Act. He went on to caution the government that it was not clear to him that Section 504 of the Rehabilitation Act authorized the government to reach so far into such a sensitive area of moral and ethical concerns.

The Court concluded:

> This regulation cannot be sustained. It is arbitrary and capricious. There may well be defects in medical procedures and hospital policies governing treatment of seriously disabled newborns in some hospitals. More fundamentally, the rising public debate over the role of physicians and family members in the difficult and sensitive situation where life may hang in the balance has raised issues which must eventually be faced at either the local or national level. The solution does not, however, lie in a hasty, ill-considered "hotline" informer rule. Government intervention into the difficult medical and human decisions that must be made in the delivery rooms and newborn intensive care units of our hospitals involves a profound change in the manner in which these decisions affecting the quality of life are made. Any intervention by an agency of the Federal Government should obviously reflect caution and sensitivity, given the present absence of a clear congressional direction. At the minimum, wide public comment prior to rulemaking is essential. Only by preserving this democratic process can good intentions be tempered by wisdom and experience.

The government, after the District Court's opinion and the Federal Court of Appeal's refusal to stay the lower court's order, issued new *proposed* regulations on July 5, 1983.[16]

Clearly, the new proposed regulations will keep the issues and controversy open. The new regulations impose the same federal procedural role in investigating complaints; the hotline remains open; and "Baby Doe Squads" will be activated upon receipt of complaints. One important change and improvement in the regulations is an acknowledgment that medical judgment can decide that in the "hopeless" case, useless therapy need not be initiated to prolong the dying process. This change does clarify somewhat the vagueness and confusion of the earlier proposed regulations. However, the debate will continue in these subjects whether or not final and effective regulations are issued.

REFERENCES

1. Prosser: Law of Torts, 3rd ed. 1964.
2. Arterburn: The Origin and First Test of Public Callings. U Penn Law Rev 75:411, 1927.
3. Schloendorff v Society of New York Hospital, 211 NY 125, 105 NE 92, 1914. Overruled on other grounds, Bing v Thunig, 2 NY 2nd 656, 143 NE 2nd 3, 163 S 2nd 3, 1957.
4. Natanson v Kline, 186 Kan 393, 350 P 2nd 1093, 1960.
5. This legal right parallels recently gained rights of female patients in areas such as abortion and sterilization.
6. A very substantial majority of the states now recognize the doctrine in one form or another and are at least in agreement concerning the elements which are essential in informing patients.
7. Crouch v Most, 78 NM 406, 432 P 2nd 250, 1967.
8. Putensen v Clay Adams, Inc., 12 Cal App 3rd 1062, 91 Cal Rptr 319, 1970.
9. Salgo v Leland Stanford Jr Univ Bd of Trustees, 154 Cal App 2nd 560, 317 P 2nd 170, 1957.
10. Canterbury v Spence, 464 F 2nd 772, DC Cir 1972, at 788.
11. In re Quinlan, 70 NJ 10, 355 A 2nd 647, 1976.
12. In re Cicero, 421 NYS 2nd 965, NY Sup Ct, 1979.
13. State v Daniels, No 81-015577 F Jol, Dade County Ct, Fla, June 23, 1981.
14. Guardianship of Philip Becker, No 1, Civil 53419, Cal App First Appellate District, Oct 19, 1981.
15. American Academy of Pediatrics, National Association of Children's Hospitals and Related Institutions. Children's Hospital National Medical Center v Margaret M Heckler, Secretary, Department of Health and Human Services, CA No 83-0774, April 14, 1983.
16. 48 Fed Reg 30846, July 5, 1983.

SECTION SIX FURTHER READINGS

1. Glasstone S, Dolan P: The Effects of Nuclear Weapons. US Department of Defense and US Department of Energy, 1977.
2. Gross B, Gross R: The Children's Rights Movement. New York, Anchor Press/Doubleday, 1977.
3. Holder A: Legal Issues in Pediatrics and Adolescent Medicine. New York, John Wiley & Sons, 1977.
4. Office of Technology Assessment, United States Congress: The Effects of Nuclear War. US Government Printing Office, 1979.
5. President's Commission for the Study of Ethical Problems in Medicine and Biomedical and Behavioral Research: Making Health Care Decisions. A Report on the Ethical and Legal Implications of In-

formed Consent in the Patient-Practitioner Relationship. Washington, DC, US Government, 1982.
6. Shannon TA, Manra JA: Law and Bioethics. Texts with Commentary on Major US Court Decisions. Ramsey, NJ, Paulist Press, 1982.

Index